C000151359

This book is not intended as a substitut(
advice of physicians. The reader should r(
physician in matters relating to his/her health and particularly
with respect to any symptoms that may require diagnosis or
medical attention.

ISBN: 978-0-9934700-0-4

First published in the UK in November 2015 by:
Seeking Sense and Science Ltd.
Bluebell Cottage, High Street, Stroud, GL6 8DR

Email address: seekingsenseandscience@gmail.com

Cover illustration by Gus Russell
Printed by Wealden Print, TN18 4QT UK

To my parents:
For their patience and enthusiasm. For listening to me for
hours as I verbalised and consolidated all I was reading and
discovering, and for their robust questioning.

To my husband:
For his patience and for helping me have the time to embark
on my journey of discovery.

INDEX

CHAPTER ONE - WHERE WE ARE TODAY

CHAPTER TWO - EXPOSING OUR MISTAKES

CHAPTER THREE - ENDING THE GLOOM EMPOWERED BY EVOLVING & TRADITIONAL KNOWLEDGE

CHAPTER ONE
WHERE WE ARE TODAY

1. WHERE WE ARE TODAY

- Overfed and undernourished
- Confused and misinformed
- Over medicated
- Intoxicated
- Suffering chronic body inflammation
- Suffering weakened immunity
- Disconnected from our bodies
- Forgotten basic knowledge for better nutrition and health
- Facing chronic disease,
- Illness and
- Mental decline

Where We Could Be

- Lean and toned
- Energetic and focused
- Happy and calm
- Healthy
- Mentally agile
- Less fretful of disease
- Higher expectations of well being into old age
- Better informed
- We could be thriving instead of just surviving

2. ARE WE ON THE BRINK OF A FOOD REVOLUTION?

Are we about to witness a food revolution? Most of what we have been advised about food over the past 70 years is being turned on its head. In America hundreds of type 2 diabetics are being cured of their diabetes by throwing existing dietary guidelines out of the window. Those with this so-called progressive disease are reversing their condition by shifting the focus towards insulin resistance as the cause.(1)

Sugar, fats, carbohydrates and proteins are being re-evaluated in dramatic fashion and the view on these food groups is changing for many reasons, not least for our new understanding of how these foods feed the good and the bad bugs in our gut that have such an impact on our health. Importantly, there is also a resurfacing understanding of how truly toxic sugar can be.

We have the internet to thank for this because through this medium very many scientists, researchers and doctors have been able to communicate their experiences. Their experiences do not relate at all to many established dietary guidelines and they are finding they are not alone.

Has a spell been broken, where we were once all much greater believers in the power of the magic bullet created in pharmaceutical laboratories – tablets and pills to fix everything? Now we are starting to look around us and witnessing the car crash that is the health of our nation ... yes living longer, but in what shape and with what prospects? Common sense may be prevailing over the reliance on false promises. The discussion of what has happened to food is becoming more sophisticated and more interesting than it ever has been. People are waking up from a slumber that has lasted several decades, during which time we have lost control of our food and relied too heavily on more and more pills.

This book is about taking our health into our own hands and embarking on our own fact finding missions to decide for ourselves what is right and what is wrong for we may well be following the wrong advice.

3. WITHIN A WHISPER OF TRIGGERING ILLNESS

The power we have over our health through what we put in our mouths should not be underestimated – the good choices and the bad ones.

Until recently we were led to believe that the DNA we are born with predetermined our health and illnesses. That having certain genes would make it inevitable that sooner or later they would kick in and we would become ill.

Today we have cause to feel far more empowered and in control of our health. We are discovering through a science known as "Epigenetics" that the food we eat and the lifestyles we choose to lead will have a direct effect on how the vast majority of our genes behave.(2)

We overdo it, don't get enough sleep, eat badly and are within a whisper of triggering illness … but re-establishing a healthy routine with an eye on food, sleep, exercise and stress can not only keep us on the path of good health but restore health as well.

My Own Story – Briefly

I came to the whole subject of nutrition, like many others now in the field, by my own health issues and the subsequent way I was dealt with by the established medical community.

I was diagnosed in 2009 with Rheumatoid Arthritis. Though my doctors successfully treated my severe symptoms, they did not offer me a cause or a cure. I was expected to carry on taking strong and potentially harmful medication for the rest of my life.

I had to find the answer to causes and possible cures myself, as to why my body had turned on me in such a dramatic, painful and life debilitating way.

4

4. ANSWERS WITH ADDED VALUE

I did find answers and along the way I found improvement and solutions to many other aspects of my health, including:

Fatigue, mood swings, anxiety and lack of concentration I rediscovered a sense of calm, energy and achievement. For it would seem that when you heal, you heal ... it is not a selective process.

Six years on and so very, very many questions later, I have collated the eye-opening information I have gathered so as to represent it in a more user-friendly form.

So much of what I have read has been buried in books and long articles that most of us may not have the time or inclination to navigate. I hope that more people may also have the chance to make my interesting journey by reading this book.

Why Should You Read What I Have To Say?

Growing up I was strongly influenced by my father. He worked from home and innovated and developed technology in a number of different industries. With a degree in chemical engineering from Imperial College, London, he is an avid reader and researcher. Annoyingly, when I was growing up, he was very partial to extensive monologues (that hasn't changed)!

Without realising it, for years, I was absorbing information on many topics but more importantly I was absorbing an attitude towards information, questioning, analysis and scientific reasoning that was relentlessly being drummed into me. I have noticed that the more scientifically trained an individual is the less they are likely to talk in absolute terms. Beware of emphatic phrases! …. Though I am sure I am guilty of it myself ….

5. GETTING ILL, BLACK HOLES AND FLAT EARTHERS

I embraced the topic of nutrition as a self-educator. Self-education is a privilege more available to us today through the internet. However the internet is a mix of incredible access to knowledge but potentially a black hole to information as there is so much of it and often very conflicting.

So we need to be wary of 'facts'. We have been dished up so many over the years that then go on to be overturned.

We need to question everything and be mindful when finding the same fact repeated endlessly on the internet; it does not make it necessarily true. It is essential to go back to basics. In this book I have attempted to find researchers, scientists and experienced clinicians who have done exactly that.

As self-educators the trick, often, is finding the right questions to ask and being mindful of how the questions are posed. For example: Why are potatoes good for us? Or why are potatoes bad for us? Can lead you down two very different routes.

The whole subject of health is in such a state of flux, disagreement and confusion. In fact it shows us that it is still possible for scientific opinion to be as divided and dogmatic as it was at the time when there were those who believed the world to be flat and others who believed it to be round. Fat, protein, carbohydrates and whole grains are fine examples of where fervent, 'religious' division of opinions can lie. Everything is being questioned.

Opening Our Minds to a Bigger Picture

We need to stand back and look at a much bigger picture to understand what is impacting on our well being and even our weight. We need to pay attention to the effects of medication, environmental toxins, stress, sleep and eating habits because they are having far more significant consequences on our bodies than we may have realised. For example how many 'bottles' of products do you have in your house? In your kitchen? (It seems you need at least five different products just for your dishwasher!) In your bathroom? (Cleaning, washing, cosmetics, grooming …) We are sold substance after substance by the marketing men. Our bodies are dealing with more chemicals than ever before. What other chemicals are we subjected to in our home and work environments, in our cars and in all the goods that we purchase?

I'm No Earth Mother But …

I don't think anyone I know would describe me as an "Earth mother". Yet my journey of discovery has led me to realise we need to claw back a closeness to nature in every way we can, in a world that is moving in the opposite direction. We did not evolve to exist in the chemical, plastic, antiseptic, sprayed environment we live in today, removed from nature, fresh, fresh food and limited exposure to sunlight and soil.

There is a balance that we have lost between protecting ourselves from, and interacting with, the bacterial world around us.

When we are exposed to bacteria we pick up the good and the bad. If we feed ourselves correctly, we feed the good bacteria what it needs. This will enhance our immunity and protect us from the bad bacteria that we are inevitably exposed to as well. So through exposure and good eating habits, we can build up our immune systems and be strong. Instead we have sterilised our immediate environments, sealed the windows, chosen to consume poor food and become weak.

Our bodies work flat out to metabolise and 'deal' with the chemicals that we let in, through medication, cosmetics, junk food, pollution, plastics and chemicals emanating from the world that surrounds us. The ammunition that our bodies need to counteract this assault takes the form of minerals, vitamins, polyphenol phytonutrients and fibre available, in good part, from fresh fruit and vegetables.

So we must eat well not only to have the nutrients we need to enhance our bacterial immunity but also to protect us from the external assault of chemicals and

7

toxins and finally with what goodness is left over, to enable our bodies to function well so that we, in turn, can feel well and energetic.

Understanding the impact of food, good and bad is one of the most powerful weapons we have to deal with the challenges. Our bodies are extremely clever and adaptable given the right ammunition. Science is beginning to understand that "we are our bugs" and that bacteria are the most adaptable life form on the planet … so there is hope. We need to adapt more intelligently to the world around us.

If we do not engage, we may find that we will continue to be manipulated and unwisely served by the food and pharmaceutical industries that have our money and not necessarily our well being in mind. All along expecting us to happily put in our mouths what they produce.

6. EMPOWERMENT

When We Really Understand Why Something Is Bad For Us
We Are More Likely To Do The Right Thing

Based on the findings of a wide variety of scientists, experienced clinicians and health writers that I have studied, I believe that there is a lot more we can do for ourselves to enhance our well being than is necessarily being offered to us by doctors, pharmaceuticals, policy makers, public authorities and institutions, big business, marketing men and the media.

We need to ask more pertinent questions about our own on-going health. We need to simplify our daily lives and reject many 'products' we do not need.

I am now off all medication, despite my specialist's advice, and have been symptom free for 4 years. I have adopted the positive recommendations in this book and have eliminated most of the negative aspects also listed. I am happier, calmer and healthier than I have been in years.

Aiming to be less fretful of disease, living a mentally and physically agile life.

Reclaiming Lost Wisdom

Not only our food but our habits and attitudes need to be reassessed. One of the reasons family is so important is for that continuity of basic knowledge that can be passed down the generations. There is much wisdom that is being lost as the modern world, in all its rush and excitement, is veering off course.

Giving our body the nutritional help it needs significantly enhances our ability to repair. Indeed if we feed ourselves properly we can exit the fog created by poor lifestyle and have the energy to achieve a whole lot more ....

Living A Long Life In Good Shape

With all the information flying around these days we think we are so well informed but so much of it is contradictory. Are we well informed? Most of us think we know the simple changes we need to make to get fit and healthy - but do we? When we do attempt to make healthy changes are we even making the right ones?

I suppose we would start with trying to eat our "five a day" but we have deviated so far down a road of poor and harmful eating habits that we are expecting those well travelled five little fruits and veg to accomplish rather a lot!

CHAPTER TWO
EXPOSING OUR MISTAKES

1. OVERFED AND STARVING – HOW DID WE MANAGE IT?

- Many of us are constantly consuming whilst failing to feed our bodies.
- We are surrounded by food that is advertised as 'healthy' but isn't.
- We are surrounded by the constant temptation of junk food.
- For all the money that is spent on processed food, it does not serve us well.
- Processed food is generally nutrient poor and high in sugar and low in fibre.
- Processed food can be so tampered with that our body no longer recognises it as food or knows what to do with it.
- We are living in a complex and profit driven world where finding and preparing fresh, wholesome food is increasingly difficult.
- The way we eat today slows down our physical and mental agility.
- We feel we do not have the time or energy to prepare food from scratch.

It's a vicious circle

… And to those out there that have been dieting for decades there has to be a reversal of mind set from:

Food is bad   "it makes me fat"
To
Food is good   "it makes me feel good and protects me from disease"

2. THE AGE OF CONVENIENCE

The expression "we want our cake and eat it too" is possibly appropriate for western society.

We have signed up for all the products of convenience. Fast food when we are out and about, pre-prepared meals when we are at home. An army of sprays and chemicals to make cleaning super easy. An army of grooming products to allow us to keep going for 24 hours plus without washing! We have an expectation of jetting off on sunny holidays. We want the latest gadgets. We work our socks off to buy all these things.

The adverts show us how we can do this .... For even though we started our day tired, after a bad night's sleep reading our tablet for too long or watching telly too late ... Even though we had a fairly mediocre lunch that has not given us much nutritional sustenance ... Even though towards the end of the day we have a splitting headache... Even though we have a social get together over drinks this evening and we really do not feel great .... We know that it doesn't matter and we can just keep going because the marketing men have told us that the pharmaceutical guys are thinking about us. They've got this great medication that you can pop into your mouth that will give you "targeted" and "fast-action" "relief". So you can slip the pack of magic back into your pocket and stride off confident that you can now manage an evening of .... Indulgence.

In the age of convenience this 'patch up' approach to mask the nasty side effects of the error of our ways is also taking place in our industrialised livestock farming, hence the ever increasing use of antibiotics in rearing animals.

According to the Soil Association "In the UK, nearly 45% of all antibiotics are used in farming, mostly used as a pharmaceutical crutch to compensate for disease-inducing conditions of factory farming, where thousands of animals are typically kept crowded together in confined spaces."

"Every inappropriate use of antibiotic in animals is potentially signing a death warrant for a future patient" Sir Liam Donaldson, former Chief Medical Officer

3. OVER MEDICATED

Western society literally chomps its way through a mountain of medication such as aspirin, ibuprofen, steroids, paracetamol, antacids, statins, painkillers, antidepressants, antibiotics, etc, etc that can leave us, often, with more problems than we set out with.

We run faster and faster in ever decreasing circles, created by modern living. Instead of trying to take back control that requires will power and self-discipline. We succumb to the following:
- Stress
- Indulging in the wrong foods
- Lack of sleep and exercise.
- Our bodies try to put the brakes on with symptoms that warn us we need to slow down or change our ways.
- Our response is to go to the doctor or the chemist and seek a magic bullet in the form of medication.
- We want something that takes immediate effect.
- The medication masks our symptoms.
- We do not modify our behaviour.
- We simply carry on.
- Until the symptoms get worse and we go back to the doctor.

Sinking In A Sea Of Low Level Illness

Every time we put something in our mouths it should be something to help our bodies, not leave us worse off, be it medication or food.

The quantity of sugared food, refined carbohydrates and much of the processed food we eat causes us:

Bloating	Reflux	Flatulence	Diarrhoea	Pain
Headaches	Cramps	Lethargy	Fatigue	Constipation
Increased Weight	Depression	Mental Issues		

AND a Weakened Immunity to Infection, Disease and Cancer

Preventable

So much of this is preventable. One day this word will become the mantra of all our family doctors but there is no time to do more than patch a patient's symptom with medication. Patients need to be advised how to prevent the symptoms from happening again. Our over-worked doctors are sinking in a sea of preventable low-level illness that, unfortunately, goes on to become more serious disease.

Our bodies have the capacity to heal and perform amazingly given the right help and care. There are some very basic steps that most of us can take to radically increase our chances of improved and excellent on-going health.

Sleep Walkers

We have chosen to mask the symptoms of our bad habits with ever-stronger medications. Even basic paracetamol is consumed by us and given to our children far too readily. We have been sleep walking around the key issues that affect our health for several decades. Today there is more cause for concern for their cumulative effect. These key issues have to be addressed with urgency as I elaborate on in the following pages:

- *We are over medicated*
- *Sugar is doing so much more harm than we realise*
- *Fat is causing serious confusion leading us to make potentially harmful choices: including the relentless demonization of saturated fats leading to ill-advised substitutes.*
- *We no longer eat in a way that gives us the vital nutrients we need*

We need to fully appreciate:
- *How bad stress is*
- *How important good sleep patterns are*
- *How vital good exercise routines are to our on-going health …. Nothing extreme, simply routine.*

4.   SUGAR UNWRAPPED

Sugar And Disease

If we don't wake up to the harm sugar is causing it has the potential to bankrupt our health service.

Worse though is what sugar, in the quantities it is consumed in today, is doing to our children. It is our duty to protect our children and we are not. In the US there are 60,000 children with diabetes. Childhood diabetes is a new and growing condition. Statistical 'bad news' data is impressively worse when it comes to nutrition in America. In the UK today the public health situation may not be as bad but in most things our tendency is to follow America's trend.

Sugar needs to be treated as public enemy number 1. Our consumption and addiction to sugar is causing suffering on a grand scale.

Americans in 2012 on average consumed over 18 times more sugar than they did in 1822 from just over 3Kg per year to 60Kg per year(3)

There are many statistics for the increase of sugar consumption over the last 100 years or so. They are all dramatic but we can see it for ourselves in the western world. Just look at the quantity of fast food and sweet snacks and drinks available and advertised all around us, all the time.

Sugar Is a Major Cause of "Metabolic Syndrome" But What Is It?

According to the National Health nhs.uk, 1 in 4 people have metabolic syndrome in the UK and Diabetes.co.uk note that it is becoming increasingly common. In the US, according to the International Diabetes Federation 1 in 3 have metabolic syndrome.

Metabolic syndrome is a collection of symptoms, caused by progressive insulin resistance, that are high risk factors for heart attack and strokes. Whether or not we appear healthy and thin very many of us have some level of metabolic syndrome already:

High Blood Pressure Abdominal Obesity
Raised Blood Sugars   Fatty Liver
Raised Blood Triglycerides
(fats in blood from sugar and refined carbohydrates)

Metabolic syndrome can eventually lead to:

Diabetes	Dementia	Kidney Failure
Heart Attacks	Mood Swings	Blindness
Strokes	Cancer	Rheumatoid Arthritis
Depression	Alzheimer's	Impotence
Infertility	Sleep Disruption	Lethargy & Fatigue
Multiple Sclerosis	Atherosclerosis	Autoimmune Disorders
Inflammatory Bowel Disease [4]		

Our Energy Overload

One of the best descriptions I have heard for why we get metabolic syndrome diseases is simply due to 'energy overload'. We are essentially eating way more sugary and sugar forming food than we can possibly metabolise efficiently and it is leading us down a path of ill-health.

Understand, Fear and Prevent "Insulin Resistance" – a Path to Dementia

When we eat sugary and processed carbohydrate foods the body responds by creating insulin in order to enable the energy of these foods to enter the cells. Unfortunately the more sugary drinks, sugar and sugar forming foods like bread and pasta we have the more insulin we produce. Our cells slowly reach a point of saturation, they do not require any more energy and resist the insulin that is still knocking on its cell door wanting to bring in more sugar/energy. This is the beginning of insulin resistance. The unwanted sugar remains outside the cells, in the bloodstream thus elevating our blood sugar levels, leading to abdominal fat and/or internal fat storage and a whole host of possible health problems including dementia(12a).

We Do Not Have to be Obese to Have Metabolic Syndrome

Metabolic syndrome starts in childhood and can progress silently and undiagnosed and is the precursor to many, many modern and increasingly prevalent conditions as mentioned. In some the fat accumulation is not necessarily external so they may appear 'thin' but this is deceptive as they may be storing fat around their internal organs instead which is extremely dangerous for on-going health.

Why Do We Still Have Vending Machines in Hospitals and Schools?

We must protect our children. We need to educate them on the dangers of sugar and stop even more people from making the same mistakes.

Vending machines full of sugary snacks and canned drinks should be removed from all schools and hospitals and people educated to truly understand the consequences of their own actions.

In our addictive haze we seem unable to prevent more children falling into the deadly trap of Metabolic Syndrome and obesity. There is no one to counteract the advertising offensive "sugar is wonderful" that enters our homes through our TVs every day.

Sugar, Fructose, Fruit – Sorting Out The Confusion

ATTENTION!!

SUCROSE is commonly known as:
Table Sugar   Natural Sugar
Sugar Cane   Sugar Beet

All SUCROSE is made up of
One part Glucose and one part FRUCTOSE

Why Highlight the Above So Carefully?

Just because something is 'natural' does not mean it is safe.
Fructose in our sugar is a very powerful disruptor of our metabolism
that needs to be understood; for sugar is put in everything these days,
even when we least expect it.

Fructose disrupts the hormones that control our normal appetite signals. This disruption can create a loss in the ability to feel full AND gives us a constant feeling of hunger that will inevitably affect the weight we put on or that we are unable to lose.[5]

Not all calories are metabolised equally. **Fructose can be converted to energy at a much faster rate than glucose.** This energy, if not used is metabolised by the liver and simply stored as fat.

Fructose is metabolised almost exclusively by the liver and our overconsumption of sugar is a heavy load for this organ. This overload triggers a hormonal imbalance that leads to metabolic syndrome, obesity, lethargy and chronic disease.

Leaving Fructose Aside Briefly – What About Glucose?

Glucose on the other hand can be metabolised by every single cell in the body but it needs insulin to be assimilated into the cells. If there is a constant overload of glucose, the body responds by producing high levels of insulin but eventually the cells start to ignore the insulin and become resistant to it (insulin resistance). By not accepting the glucose into the cells, sugar remains in the blood leading to high blood sugar levels and this state can eventually lead to type 2 diabetes and a whole host of other health issues. This process continues with the addition of refined carbohydrates in the diet, leading to further insulin resistance.

The Rise and Rise of Fructose Consumption Has Lead to the Increase in Metabolic Syndrome

The adding of sugar to our food over several decades whether the dreaded processed sugar High Fructose Corn Syrup or simply ordinary table sugar (from natural sugar cane or sugar beet) has meant that our fructose consumption has rocketed. Fructose is being added to all our processed foods, be they sweet or savoury and most especially to food labelled 'low fat', as sugar is used to replace the taste lost when fat is removed.

Fructose Has Gone From Being A Fundamental Survival Tool To A Killer Due To Our Overconsumption

The link between metabolic syndrome and fructose is a fundamental survival mechanism that exists in the animal kingdom and was of great importance to our ancestors' survival in the winter months. ….

Fascinating research in America is putting a new slant on fructose and is concluding that one of the initial symptoms of metabolic syndrome, insulin resistance was once *"a normal process not a disease"*. In fact metabolic syndrome is a *"fat storage condition"* essential to the animal kingdom but a precursor to disease for us, in our world today.[6]

The research points out that fructose enables animals to readily lay down fat stores in their bodies to see them through the winter months.

For example take the hibernating bear .....

Why Bears Have A Sweet Tooth

Bears load up with fructose in the autumn prior to hibernation enabling them to lay down and store substantial, additional fat to normal. They will consume vast quantities of sweet berries and fruits in the autumn that will contain greater amounts of fructose than earlier in the year when the fruits are less ripe.

This continuous and increased consumption of fructose 'triggers' what is effectively metabolic syndrome: insulin resistance, raised fats in their blood, increased abdominal fat, fatty liver and reduced energy levels, all important for their survival through the winter hibernation.

Birds That Fly South in the Winter Load Up with Fructose

Migratory birds increase their fructose consumption so that they can increase their bodies' fat deposits to allow them to survive the long, non-stop flights to sunnier climates.

But Animals Stop Consuming And
Humans Just Carry On

The Bears And Birds Burn It Off

In the animal kingdom however the bear effectively fasts over the winter months and the migratory birds burn their fat off during their long, non stop, flights and by the time the spring comes the bear will be lean again.

Humans however, through their ever increasing consumption of fructose have triggered the 'fat switch' activated insulin resistance and metabolic syndrome but continue to feast on sugar all year round and make their condition even worse by their over consumption of refined carbohydrates as well.

Thus fructose will then continue to be turned into fat in the body, stored and accumulated around the vital organs of a 'thin' person and <u>additionally</u> as belly fat in an obese person. (For further details read "The Fat Switch" by Doctor Richard Johnson.)

Spotlight On The Average Modern Western Diet

Should we be that surprised so many are estimated to have metabolic syndrome?

Breakfast's Loaded Sugar and Carb Opportunity
Cereals – Bread – Jam – Pastries – Fruit Juice
Mid Morning Snack's Loaded Sugar and Carb Opportunity
Biscuits – Cake – Chocolate Bars - Coffee or Tea with Sugar – Fizzy Drinks - Crisps

Lunch's Loaded Sugar and Carb Opportunity
Fast Food - Sandwiches – Bread – Crackers – Fruit Juice – Fizzy Drinks - Crisps

Mid Afternoons Loaded Sugar and Carb Opportunity
Crisps – Chocolate Bars – Fizzy Drinks – Dried Fruit

Supper's Loaded Sugar and Carb Opportunity
Pizza - Pasta – Noodles – Rice – Condiments eg ketchup or mayonnaise – Sugar loaded Pre-prepared Meals – Ice Cream – Fizzy Drinks/Alcohol

… And Even the Super Evil Late Evening Snack
Cereal – Chocolate – Biscuits – Hot Sugared Drink

Like a YoYo

With feeding patterns like this or similar we are increasing our blood sugars and disrupting our hormones, leading us to feel the need to be in perpetual 'grazing mode', trying to maintain a sugar high so that we don't feel bad. (Headaches, lethargy, anxiety, etc).

Snacking is the curse of our time, it has lead to a constant flow of sugars and carbohydrates into our body.

THE AMAZING POWER OF FRUCTOSE THAT WE MUST TAME

Fructose Does Not Suppress the "I'm Hungry" Signal (Ghrelin Hormone)

Ghrelin is the hormone that is responsible for giving feelings of hunger. Fructose in sugar will not allow it to be suppressed. So we can continue consuming and remain hungry.(7)

Fructose Suppresses the "I'm Full" Signal Peptide YY
(and why it is important to eat slowly)

It is important to know that the "I'm hungry" hormone Ghrelin, found in the stomach is not responsible for telling us when we are full.(8) That is left to another hormone that is found further down in the intestine and is known as Peptide YY. This hormone kicks in about 20 minutes after we start eating. This time delay is the reason why it is important to eat slowly. If we finish our dish in 10 minutes and want seconds ... wait 10 minutes ... then decide.

Fructose Disrupts Leptin Signalling – Leading Our Body to Think It Is Starving When In Fact It Is Overweight

Leptin is a hormone discovered in the 1990s that is formed in the fat cells, so the more fat cells we have the more leptin we have. It is responsible for signalling to the brain that we have enough energy stored in our fat cells.(9) In this situation we will not feel hungry, we will feel energetic and well. The body can afford to be 'liberal' with its energy stores. We feel energized and on top of the world .... Beautiful when all the hormones are in balance ....

However leptin, like insulin, suffers from being ignored by the body when levels get too high. So when more and more fat accumulates in the body, especially through on-going sugar consumption, more and more leptin is produced. This continual production of leptin leads to leptin resistance. In other words, even though leptin is being produced the brain starts to ignore its signals.

Thus, despite the fact that you are putting on weight and eating plenty of food all the time, the brain, because it is not accepting the signals, believes it is in starvation mode.

The body therefore believes it needs to conserve energy. This gives the feeling of sluggishness and lack of desire to do physical activity. This preference for inactivity is a symptomatic characteristic of obesity. Believing itself to be starving, the body is not so willing to burn its fat stores.

Restoring the hormonal balance that sugar disrupts is key and when achieved it is possible to restore good health, an ideal weight and increased vitality.

Fructose Takes its Toll on the Liver

As mentioned when we consume sucrose (table sugar) the glucose molecules are able to be metabolised by every single cell in the body. The fructose molecule however can only be metabolised by the liver. When we consume too much sugar the liver becomes overloaded and instead of breaking it down it stores it as extra liver fat.

Looking after the liver is crucial. It is the body's major fat burning organ and regulates fat metabolism. Eating a high fibre diet is fundamental to health and weight loss as it slows down digestion and gives a feeling of fullness. To illustrate this take the example of a glass of freshly squeezed orange juice. It may easily contain the juice of four oranges. Drinking one glass of orange juice is quick but one would struggle to consume four whole oranges … and without the fibre in the juice the fructose is rapidly metabolised by the liver and converted to fat.[10]

The 'Speed' of Fructose Intake

A can of a sweet fizzy drink will, on average have 10 teaspoons of sugar. The rate and quantity at which these are consumed is one of the main driving forces of obesity in the young.

Sports Drinks promoted as healthy are often, simply sugared water of some form and can be just as harmful. These drinks also have the ability, due to the presence of fructose and absence of fibre, to be converted into fat in the body with great speed.

Fructose and Diabetes

According to the American paediatric endocrinologist Dr Robert Lustig and author of "Fat Chance", if you eat an extra 150 calories a day of healthy whole foods your risk of diabetes is not affected. If, however, you increase your calories by 150 per day by consuming a sugary drink then your risk of developing diabetes goes up 11 fold. Lustig maintains that calories from other sources can lead to weight gain, calories from sugar uniquely contribute to the risk of type 2 diabetes. Dr Lustig has studied the dangers of fructose and is one of the loudest voices in America, warning of those dangers.

Addiction To Fructose

It is said that sugar is as addictive as cocaine, as it triggers the release of dopamine in the brain, and is not easy to 'come off' but after a few days to a couple of weeks the initial cravings of withdrawal diminish and it becomes easier to resist temptation. (11)

Fructose Feeds the Bad Bugs In Your Digestive Tract

Taking expensive probiotics (good bacteria) whilst still consuming large amounts of sugar may well be a waste of money as sugar will feed your bad bugs and help increase their population and prevent them from being overpowered by your good gut flora/bacteria (responsible in large part for your immune system).

…. And Finally What About Fructose in Fruit?

After reading all about fructose it wouldn't be surprising if you wanted to stay away from it altogether!

BUT whole fruit is full of very valuable antioxidants, enzymes and fibre that help reduce the effect of the fructose compared to processed foods and sweet drinks. Give up on the processed food not the fruit. Eat fruit in moderation especially when trying to lose weight and eat it when it is less ripe and its antioxidant content is higher and its fructose content is lower. Get to know which fruits are higher and lower in fructose – some examples are given further on in the book under "Juicing or Blending".

Sugar's Canon Balls - A Summary

In Summary Sugar Doesn't Just Fire One Canon Ball At Your Health

It Fires Three

Shot one triggers insulin resistance, metabolic syndrome, diabetes, external obesity and unhealthy, internal fat stores around your organs, leading on to many inflammatory diseases

Shot two feeds the pathogens (the bad bacteria in your gut) harming the balance of your good gut bacteria that, as we will go on to read, is now believed to make up a staggering 75% of your immune system

Shot three it depletes your body's store of nutrients especially minerals like magnesium needed to metabolise the sugars and carbohydrates, leaving you deficient in vital nutrients.

It's Not the Saturated Fat – It's The Sugar[11a]

We should be transplanting from deep in our psyche that image of butter-lined, clogged arteries with an image of bags of sugar transforming themselves from crystals of white purity, labelled 'fat-free' in the packaging - to fat of the worst possible kind, storing itself doggedly around our organs and our belly once we consume…. Pure evil.

Is it time to replace the "Low Fat" label with a "No Sugar" One?

Why Sweeteners Are Not a Good Idea [12]

The debate on sweeteners goes backwards and forwards but research is now showing that aspartame may raise insulin and that sweeteners in general cause the body to think it is about to receive sugar and when it doesn't it causes craving. In addition more research is needed on the effect on gut bacteria and indications are that the sweeteners may cause disruption here too.

However there is also another fundamental reason why they are not serving us well:

Sweeteners maintain our "sweet tooth". As we reduce our sugar and sweetener consumption our palate will change and we will become more sensitive to the sugar tastes, meaning that, eventually, a little bit of fruit or a tiny teaspoon tip of honey will give us plenty of sugary taste. Not, however, if we keep bombarding our palate with sweeteners.

5. WE MUST GET OUR HEADS' AROUND INSULIN RESISTANCE BEFORE WE CAN'T GET OUR HEADS' AROUND ANYTHING AT ALL!

1. In 2003 just over 10% of the UK population was diagnosed as pre-diabetic. By 2011, according to the British Medical Journal, that figure had more than tripled to over 35% of the UK population.
2. Pre-diabetes means that your cells' resistance to insulin is steadily progressing. The cells in the body are less able to metabolise glucose leading to glucose remaining outside the cells, in the bloodstream and therefore causing high blood sugar levels. Unless diet and exercise is improved type 2 diabetes will follow.
3. There is a growing belief that there is a link between type 2 diabetes and Alzheimer's. Studies show that approximately half of people with type 2 diabetes will go on to develop Alzheimer's disease leading to this condition being nicknamed "type 3 diabetes". Researchers noted that the brain of those with Alzheimer's, just like the body of those with type 2 diabetes, was progressively less able to use and metabolise glucose, a fundamental consequence of insulin resistance.
4. Insulin is crucial to trigger other chemicals in the brain and is fundamental for memory and learning. Insulin resistance will hamper these functions and lead to poorer cognitive ability, brain shrinkage and dementia.(12a)

6. INFLAMMATION – A WORD WE ALL NEED TO KNOW MORE ABOUT

What's The Big Deal With Inflammation

We need to plug on with the unsavoury facts to <u>make</u> us really address better habits.

Understanding inflammation is probably one of the most important aspects about our health to learn about in order to achieve lasting well-being.

Is Inflammation a Good or Bad Thing?
Without Inflammation Wounds And Infections Would Never Heal

But for many it is out of control, and at the root of a whole host of conditions in western or developed societies.

What Is Inflammation?

It is an important part of the body's immune response and protection.
It works in our bodies to remove harmful agents, damaged cells and starts the healing process. An obvious example is the puffy swollen skin around a cut, but this process goes on inside the body as well.

So What's the Problem?

The Inflammatory process that should be beneficial is out of control. Most of us are affected in some way by inflammation that just will not subside due to the damaging food we eat and hectic lifestyles we lead. Our bodies are continually trying to repair damage with an inflammatory response. Gradually over time the on-going inflammation will develop into some form of chronic health issue.

Inflammation is a Symptom of Many Modern Diseases.

Examples of inflammatory conditions are asthma, allergies, diabetes, heart disease, cancer, Alzheimer's and arthritis … in fact any condition ending in "it is". (colitis, rheumatoid arthritis, dermatitis, diverticulitis, etc) and much more, including brain degeneration. (13)

Inflammation is Preventable

Diet and lifestyle factors are the cause of inflammation. We all need help in finding causes and education on prevention but instead all we are offered over and over again are medications that are only able to reduce our symptoms but offer no solution.

The Relationship Between Our Gut and Inflammation and the Brain

A fascinating book called Brain Maker, published in March 2015 by Dr D Perlmutter, a neurologist and nutritionist, deals in detail with the influence of gut health in protecting our brain health. Perlmutter elaborates on how chronic inflammation and brain degeneration are closely linked. In fact he states that gut health or …

"… state of your microbiome determines whether or not your body is fanning the flames of inflammation or squelching them."

Consuming sugar will feed the bad bugs and yeast in our gut and encourage chronic inflammation. Gut dysfunction and inflammation are linked to people suffering depression, in fact, the compound serotonin, known for mood control, is mainly found in the gut.

With inflammation now starting to be viewed as possibly a primary risk factor for depression, neuroscience today is gravitating toward studying dietary changes rather than pharmaceutical prescriptions for treatment of depression.

Dr Perlmutter goes on to say *".... chronic inflammation and free radical damage are concepts that lie front and center in neuroscience today, but no pharmaceutical approach can come anywhere close to a dietary prescription for managing your intestinal bacteria."*

In his book Perlmutter takes a close look at the foods needed to protect and enhance our intestinal health and our brain and by default our health. Through pre and probiotic foods, fermented foods such as yoghurts and homemade sauerkraut, green vegetables and other low carbohydrate foods, gluten free foods and quality saturated and monounsaturated fats, oily fish for anti-inflammatory Omega 3 and vitamin D.

Know The Difference Between Acute And Chronic Inflammation

ACUTE: the body dealing with a cut to the arm is an easy example of a healthy acute inflammatory response. The tissue surrounding the cut goes red, becomes swollen and hurts as the damaged cells release chemicals that send signals to our white blood cells to come in and clean up the wound of all damaged tissue ready for other cells, collagen and cholesterol to step in and carry out repair. Once this is done the swelling subsides, the pain goes away.

CHRONIC: the body dealing with a constant intake of sugars, carbohydrates, crisps and fried foods, for example, that trigger inflammation, or constant stress that releases cortisol or lack of sleep are examples of continual attack that our bodies try to address with an inflammatory response. A response that can never subside for the attack is on-going.

This chronic cycle of repair, more inflammation, break up of repaired tissue and more repair on top of repair is the basis of atherosclerosis (otherwise known as the hardening of, or the obstruction of the arteries). This narrowing of vessels can lead on to strokes, heart attacks or reduced blood flow to the brain causing mental decline. Simultaneously to this, as mentioned, sugar consumption can trigger a host of negative chemical reactions and feed the bad bugs and yeast in our gut that all lead to and enhance our chronic inflammation.

Are You Thriving In Your Life Or Just Surviving

Lifestyle Changes to Reduce the Need for an Inflammatory Response
These 7 points are the fundamental keys to reducing inflammation and maintaining good long-term health:
- Cut out sugar and <u>unhealthy</u> fats
- Exercise
- Get healthy sun exposure for the best source of vitamin D (see page on vitamin D for details on exposure).
- Eat nutritious wholefoods
- Manage stress
- Get good sleep
- Avoid chemicals and toxins

It cannot be overstated how much of an impact those seven points have on our health, not just in terms of health or illness but in terms of the difference between merely surviving or really thriving in your life. Disruption in any one of these areas should be addressed.

Changes To Diet to Reduce and Reverse Inflammation

Avoid pro-inflammatory foods:
Processed food, sugar and polyunsaturated vegetable oils, particularly in processed food – these foods combine to flood our bodies with pro-inflammatory compounds.

The media and the general 'buzz' seems to focus on making sure we consume anti inflammatory food such as:
- Oily fish, cod liver or krill oils
- Yoghurts and fermented foods
- Foods high in anti-oxidants and phytonutrients, the compounds responsible for the rich colours and tastes in vegetables, herbs, spices and fruits.
- Foods containing vitamins B6, B12 and folic acid.

All these foods are indeed vital but maybe we are forgetting to focus equally on the food that is causing too much inflammation.

We can make a huge difference to our health by eliminating the enormous quantity of inflammatory foods that have entered our modern diet. Sugar is a primary culprit but we must also look at the very large quantity of unhealthy vegetable oils that are being used especially in processed and fast food – an overwhelming source of pro inflammatory Omega 6....

Omega 6 – One Giant Inflammatory Leap Too Far?

7. UNRAVELLING FAT

The Omega Band Wagon

Everyone has jumped onto the 'Omega Band Wagon'. How many of us, though, know anything about it? We probably take cod liver oil, fish oil or omega supplements. What do you take? Omega 3? Omega 3 & 6 combined? Omega 3, 6 & 9? Why do we take it and how much should we actually consume?

What Are Omega Essential Fatty Acids?
These are necessary for health but obtainable only through diet. In essence:

Omega 3 Acts To Reduce Inflammation
Polyunsaturated Fat
And is the only Omega that may require supplementation

Omega 6 Acts To Promote Inflammation
Polyunsaturated Fat
(Both Omega 3 and 6 are vital but should be consumed in more equal measure, Omega 6 is more readily available through dietary sources than Omega 3. Omega 6 is only required in moderate quantities for the healing process).

Omega 9 Acts To Reduce Inflammation
Monounsaturated Fat
(Not an essential fat as the body can produce it. Also abundant in olive oil.)

NB: Omega 3 is best from animal sources such as oily fish. Plant based Omega 3 requires processing by the body to benefit in the same way as animal sources but this process is not very efficient.

The Omega 3/Omega 6 Ratio

THE PROBLEM: Ideally we should consume far more equal measures of omegas. Some say a ratio of 1:4 some say 1:2(14)
BUT
Western society, more than at any other time in history, is consuming on average 20 times more pro-inflammatory omega 6 than anti-inflammatory omega 3. The ratio for many has become 1:20 even 1:25

How Are We Consuming So Much Omega 6?

In the last 150 years with the advent of industrial production of vegetable oils there has been a dramatic rise of around 10-20 times in the consumption of pro-inflammatory Omega 6 through processed and fast food, with some people consuming over 25 times more Omega 6 than Omega 3. This may well be a major reason inflammatory diseases have reached such numbers in the West.

Omega 6 Sources to Avoid and Sources to Seek

Unhealthy: Processed foods that contain inexpensive vegetable oils, such as fries, crisps, pre-prepared foods, cakes and biscuits.
Healthy: Olive oil, avocados, 'grass-fed' butter, fresh nuts and seeds that not only give you enough Omega 6 but many other beneficial nutrients.

The Problem With Vegetable And Seed Oils

These oils are called PUFAs (Polyunsaturated Fatty Acids). They are predominantly:
1. Generally very high in Pro-inflammatory Omega 6.
2. Unstable when exposed to heat and light and susceptible to being turned rancid and toxic during the heat generating, production processes in pre-prepared foods and fried food. This is how trans fats, trans-unsaturated

fatty acids or trans fatty acids are generated. They have been shown to be consistently associated with coronary heart disease.(14a)

3. Consumed in extraordinary quantities through processed food:
    Fast food, fries, crisps, cakes, biscuits, prepared meals all topped with more of the same in lashings of sauces such as mayonnaise or tomato sauce and baked produce topped with margarine.
4. Leading to chronic inflammation and disease. (14b)

In Nature Plant Oil Is Wrapped Up Tightly In Small Nuts And Seeds
Allowing Us To Only Access Its Oils In Small Healthy Quantities
Nature Did Not Mean Us To Process These Foods On A Vast Scale.

Suddenly in the Middle of the 20th Century We Were Told to Alter Our Fat Eating Habits

Have the very substances that we have been encouraged to substitute butter and animal fat for - the promotion of vegetable/seed oils, caused chronic inflammation, especially in the quantities consumed today? We have removed saturated fat that protected us from inflammation and replaced it with a form of fat that promotes inflammation. In addition by removing the same healthy saturated fats from our foods and in order to maintain the 'taste' of those foods we substituted it with another inflammatory ingredient – sugar.

When we check the labels we normally find that the 'low fat' option of a processed food will contain more sugar than the 'normal' version (check out for example the low fat and normal mayonnaise labels next time you are at the supermarket).

How Did We Fall Out of Love with Saturated Fat –
The Demonization Of Butter Time Line (15)

1. Like many things it started in America. In 1911 the first shortening product (fat to make pastry) to be mass-produced and made entirely out of vegetable oil was introduced. This was the beginning of what has become a vastly lucrative industry where vegetable oil has replaced animal fat and is to be found in most processed foods and indeed in home-cooking, as people have been told to fear butter and animal fat and replace it with heat processed plant oil and margarine.

2. By the 1920s-30s Coronary Heart Disease (CHD) was reaching epidemic levels not seen before. Doctors were finding that this 'uncommon' disease was becoming a 'common' cause of death.

3. By the 1950s doctors had forgotten a time when CHD was uncommon.

4. It should be noted that the consumption of saturated fat had always been a dietary staple amongst populations all over the world but what had changed was the incidence of heart disease in America.

5. With CHD reaching very concerning levels in the US by the 1950s scientists and government were looking for answers.

6. Into the story enters Ancel Keys, a pathologist at the University of Minnesota. A scientist who today appears on thousands of sites across the internet. Sites that vilify him for aggressively pushing his theory called the "diet-heart hypothesis", the catalyst for our fear of butter and saturated fats.

7. Ancel Keys' theory is now said to be based on very poor science. In essence he was very selective and manipulative with his findings only including results that fit with his theory and blatantly discarding the ugly facts that didn't fit into his hypothesis. He was however a very charismatic, strongly opinionated man who had good connections with influential and non-scientific individuals who accepted what he stated to be true. His public profile had gained such momentum he even had his face on the front of Time Magazine in 1961.

8. In the same year, based on Ancel Keys' work the American Heart Association published guidelines for the first time advising US citizens to reduce their intake of saturated fats.

9. By 1977 this advice became official and adopted by the US government. The rest of the western world soon followed.
10. In 1990 McDonalds replaced animal fat to cook its fries with vegetable oil.
11. The West has followed Key's hypothesis for over 60 years and during that time, despite best efforts and hundreds of millions spent to prove his theories, no one has satisfactorily proved him to be correct.
12. In the meantime and despite adopting his recommendations we have seen Coronary Heart Disease (CHD) become one of the western world's major killers.

A Tribute to John Yudkin Author of "Pure, White and Deadly"

At the time of Ancel Keys notoriety a less 'charismatic' but noteworthy scientist in England by the name of John Yudkin of Christ College Cambridge who worked at Queen Elizabeth College, London, was protesting that the problem lay with sugar and not saturated fat. He was aggressively discredited by Ancel Keys and the powerful sugar industry. In 1972 he wrote a book called "Pure, White and Deadly" in America it was called "Sweet and Dangerous" and had success worldwide. The last paragraph of Chapter 1 begins 'I hope that when you have read this book I shall have convinced you that sugar is really dangerous.'

In 2009 an endocrinologist, interested in childhood obesity, by the name of Dr Robert Lustig recorded a lecture called 'Sugar – The Bitter Truth'. This lecture has been viewed many millions of times on You Tube. In it he revealed his own independent research on sugar came to the same conclusions as Yudkin. He noted his admiration of Yudkin's work and "Pure, White and Deadly" was republished for the second time in 40 years in 2012. Dr Robert Lustig has published the book "Fat Chance: The Hidden Truth About Sugar, Obesity and Disease".

Butter is Wonderful

Butter has created so much confusion and anxiety in people in the past few decades. Let's try to dispel the fear of butter and also encourage its celebration as a valuable nutritional tool. One that most of us love to eat!

For centuries cultures around the globe have valued and celebrated butter for its health benefits, cultures whose knowledge and observation of food was passed down from generation to generation unchanged.

Butter Offers a Perfect Tool For Bringing Vitamins and Minerals Together

Fat soluble vitamins work closely with minerals found in vegetables. Adding butter to your steamed vegetables is an easy daily dish that will bring vital nutrients together in an easily absorbable way. Butter offers fat soluble vitamins A, D, E, K2 and assists the absorption of important trace minerals: Chromium, Copper, Manganese, Selenium and Zinc.

So Put Butter On Your Vegetables!

…. A Note on Quality: In order to obtain the many health benefits of butter the quality of the cow's diet is vital. Pasture/grass fed cows produce healthy, nutrient rich yellow/orange butter (beta-carotene from the grass). Corn fed cows will not offer the same goodness and their butter is whiter and waxy. The richer the pasture the cow feeds on the more nutritious the butter. In the summer and autumn butter will be at its best.

…. And a Note of Caution: The Real Danger of Butter
So you have been told you can have butter after all – but what are you going to do with it? The fact is we love to pile butter onto carbs! Toast, crumpets, muffins, sandwiches, cakes, none of which are very healthy.

Does Anyone Want To Hear About The Benefits Of Saturated Fats!

To say it is a little bit irritating is an understatement …. But now that we are beginning to be told that saturated fat is good, especially butter and grass-fed animal fat that have been denied us for so long, it will not be surprising if most of us throw down the towel and scream for someone to make up their minds!

Well it has well and truly started. Testimonials abound from heart surgeons to research scientists to doctors who have been recommending a low saturated fat diet for decades and are now saying that the advice that has been given was wrong. Now a growing consensus believe:

- Saturated fat is not the cause of our modern diseases but it actually plays many important roles in the body chemistry (15a)
- Saturated fat is stable to cook with compared to polyunsaturated fats (see fats comparison chart at the end of this section).
- It's good for our heart, raising our so-called good HDL cholesterol. (16)
- Saturated fats and the effect on dietary cholesterol can help prevent anxiety and mood swings and even violence, that lead to unhealthy effects of stress. (17)
- It promotes a healthy immune system. (15a)
- It promotes healthy bones. (15a)
- Saturated fat makes up at least 50% of the cell membranes providing their necessary stiffness and integrity. (15a)
- Omega-3 fatty acids are better retained in the tissues when the diet is rich in saturated fats.(15a)
- Your brain needs saturated fat to fully function and in addition has the added benefit of stimulating the growth of new brain cells. (18)
- Saturated fat can affect particle size of LDL cholesterol that can influence proneness to heart disease. (15a)

SOME POINTS TO REFLECT ON WITH REGARDS TO CHOLESTEROL

When It Comes to Cholesterol Size Matters

Our so-called "good" cholesterol (HDL) is responsible for sweeping away our LDL "Bad" cholesterol once the LDL has carried out its function to repair tissue damage.

Labelling LDL cholesterol "bad" cholesterol is now viewed by many as misleading as LDL performs the important function helping to repair tissue damage.

Where the issue with LDL cholesterol lies, it is argued, is in the size of the proteins that attach themselves to the cholesterol (lipids) forming what are known as Lipoprotein. The size of lipoprotein you have can depend very much on your genes, but also your lifestyle, your environment and your diet (sugar of course being particularly bad).

Large lipoproteins that attach to LDL particles are best. Then there are the very small 'dense' lipoproteins that attach to LDL particles. These are concerning for health and heart disease. Small dense LDL particles can bury themselves in the lining of your arteries, oxidise and cause inflammation and blockage over time.

So if you have the large, so called "fluffy" LDL particles you can stand easy, even if your levels of LDL are high. The trouble is, if your LDL is high you will probably be encouraged to take statins, with all their possible adverse effects, irrespective of the size of lipoprotein attached to your LDL.

The common tests we have to measure our LDL and HDL cholesterol does not look at LDL particle sizes that is the more accurate indicator of heart health. Ideally cholesterol tests should perhaps look for the protein called "Apoprotein a" that when present in the LDL cholesterol creates elevated levels of Lp(a) Lipoprotein(a). Its presence is now becoming more widely associated with higher risk for cardiovascular disease. (19)

Reduce Inflammation In Your Body To Lower Cholesterol

Reducing your risk of inflammation in the body (good food, exercise, good sleep and stress management) can help to drop the body's production of LDL cholesterol as it will not need to produce as much for repairing inflammatory damage.

Our Bodies Indicate Cholesterol's Importance By Not Only Producing but Recycling It

There are those who remind us that cholesterol is essential for the functioning of our body, especially as we get older, as it is a vital component of the body's repair mechanism. It is so important that our liver produces about 75% of our body's cholesterol and goes on to recycle it as well. It makes up our cell membranes, and is fundamental for hormone and nerve function. Our brains need up to 25% of our body's total cholesterol. It is needed to synthesise vitamin D and form cortisol, oestrogen, progesterone and testosterone. It acts as an antioxidant repairing damage in the body and is crucial in the body's ability to fight infection.

Cholesterol and Heart Attacks

New research (20) is showing that the majority of people suffering their first heart attack have normal cholesterol levels. This is in tune with what more and more cardiologist/heart surgeons are observing from their own clinical experience.

Is Cholesterol In Fact A Vital Antioxidant That We Need More Of As We Get Older?

Cholesterol functions as an antioxidant and the body increases its production when responding to external stresses and the need for the body to repair damage. Those who have reached very old age are often found to have high cholesterol levels. Levels, possibly, that are a response to the increased need for repair in the older body. (20a)

44

Testing Your Cholesterol and Other Health Check Markers

Next time you have a blood test don't just focus on cholesterol as many do, note other markers for good on-going health, they may be more informative:

- Blood tests that indicate how your **blood sugars** are behaving, for we should be more worried about our sugar intake and its effect on our bodies.

- **CRP (C Reactive Protein)** An inflammatory marker; it can give you an idea of your level of internal inflammation though it cannot determine where the inflammation is.

- A check to test for elevated **Homocysteine** levels is causing much debate at the moment. Some say it is a crucial test for cardiovascular risk. Others say not unless you have a family history of heart disease. It is not a test that is currently offered readily. However high levels of Homocysteine are associated with increased cardiovascular health in all age and ethnic groups and neurodegenerative disease. (20b)

  According to Patrick Holford who is a leading spokesman in Britain on nutrition, who has written over 30 books on health and is founder of the Institute of Optimum Nutrition: "… if you are not optimally nourished homocysteine can accumulate in the blood, increasing the risk of over 50 diseases, including heart attacks, strokes, certain cancers, diabetes, depression and Alzheimer's."

  Fortunately, Holford along with many others believe that, even though high levels of Homocysteine are common in today's society, these levels can be corrected quickly and relatively easily with the administering of B vitamins. In particular B12 (often lacking in vegetarians), B2, B6, Folate (often lacking in those who do not eat enough leafy greens) and zinc. Holford dedicates a whole chapter to this subject in his book "The Optimum Nutrition Bible".

A word of warning when it comes to taking tests … a 'not so good' result should not necessarily be a cue for more medication but a prompter for better nutrition …

45

The Story of Cholesterol and Statins - What Will Happen in the Final Scene?

The story of cholesterol and statins is still acting out. Controversy is raging.

A large section of the medical community believe that the whole issue of cholesterol and statins is based on bad science and that prescribing it to millions of people is simply turning them into "patients" who are not necessarily ill. In addition they may well suffer from a range of side affects, some of which are quite serious. They believe that for older people statins are removing the protective effect of cholesterol as people who die at an older age are more likely to have higher cholesterol.(20c)

The subject of cholesterol is a complex subject full of intrigue. If you wish to pursue it more in depth there is a list of interesting authors for you to research, listed in the reference section at the back of this book.(21)

Maybe We Should Be Shifting the Emphasis Away from Lowering LDL Cholesterol to Raising HDL Cholesterol Instead?

Additional risk factor indicators for unhealthy arteries are HDL/cholesterol ratio and triglyceride/HDL ratio. Your doctor can tell you whether your ratios are healthy. In both cases, however, increasing your HDL is positive.

How Do We Raise Our HDL Cholesterol?
- Cut out processed foods with its sugars and processed oils
- Eat whole, fresh foods, increasing your vitamin and mineral intake
- Ensure vitamin D intake is addressed (see Vitamin D section)
- Buy the best meat and dairy that is affordable
- Reduce high content omega 6 vegetable oils and avoid cooking with them
- Increase healthy fats: butter, avocados, coconut oil, unheated olive oil
- Focus on increasing omega 3 and reducing omega 6 intake (1:2 ratio)
- Look after gut health (see later section)
- Exercise, stay calm and sleep well
Do this little lot and we will benefit in many more ways than just raising our HDL!

Inflammation And Fat - Which Fats/Oils To Use

Summary

Polyunsaturated Fat – Eg Vegetable and Seed Oils
-        Generally high in Pro-Inflammatory Omega 6
-        Contain Anti-inflammatory Omega 3
-        Not stable when cooked at high temperatures eg for frying

Monounsaturated Fat – Eg Olive Oil
-        Low in Pro-Inflammatory Omega 6
-        Relatively stable when cooked at high temperatures
-        Offers health benefits if cold-pressed production methods are used and is best consumed cold.

Saturated Fat– Eg Butter, Coconut Oil, Animal Fats
-        Lowest in Pro-Inflammatory Omega 6
-        Stable when cooked
-        Solid at room temperature

Fats Highest in Saturated Fat

	Sat %	Mono Unsat %	Poly Unsat %	Omega 3 Anti Inflamm %	Omega 6 Pro Inflamm %
CoconutOil	**86.5**	5.8	1.8	-	1.8
Butter	**62.0**	29.0	4.0	0.3	2.7
Palm Oil	**49.3**	37.0	9.3	0.2	9.1
Beef Tallow	**49.8**	41.8	4.0	0.6	3.1

Fats Highest in Mono Unsaturated Fat

	Sat %	**Mono Unsat %**	Poly Unsat %	Omega 3 Anti Inflamm %	Omega 6 Pro Inflamm%
Olive Oil	13.8	**73.0**	10.5	0.8	9.8
Canola/ Rapeseed	8.0	**58.5**	29.0	5.8	23.0
Sunflower	9.0	**57.3**	29.0	-	29.0
Goose Fat	27.7	**56.7**	11.0	0.5	9.8
Duck Fat	33.2	**49.3**	12.9	1.0	11.9
Peanut Oil	16.9	**46.2**	32.0	-	32.0
Pig Lard	39.2	**45.1**	11.2	1.0	10.2
Chicken Fat	29.8	**44.7**	20.9	1.0	19.5

Fats Highest in Poly Unsaturated Fat

	Sat %	Mono Unsat %	**Poly Unsat %**	Omega 3 Anti Inflamm %	Omega 6 Pro Inflamm%
Safflower	6.2	14.4	**74.6**	-	74.6
Flaxseed	9.4	20.2	**66.0**	!53.3!	12.7
Walnut Oil	9.1	22.8	**63.3**	10.4	53.0
Soybean	15.6	22.8	**57.7**	6.8	50.4
Corn Oil	12.9	27.6	**54.7**	1.2	53.5
Sesame	14.2	39.7	**41.7**	0.3	41.3

Percentages are approximate as natural variation occurs but the figures give an important understanding of the underlying ratios. (22)

48

Will We Return To Cooking Our Fast Food Fries And Chips In Animal Fat?

It wouldn't make the vegetarians happy … but ….

Our fries from some of the biggest fast food chains were much tastier up until the 1990's when they changed from using beef tallow to vegetable oil.

We have taken a natural, essential food like animal fat or coconut oil that has been available to man and animal for all of history, that our physiology has been built up around, and suddenly replaced it in the last 70 years with something completely different and in such enormous proportions.

The scale of industry and mass production today allows, what may seem small changes to our diet, to be magnified up into proportions that can have effects that we never anticipated and the plant oil industry may be an example of this.

Even though recent revelations have helped highlight possible dangers of vegetable oils with adverse publicity about 'trans fats' and 'hydrogenated oils' we have not tackled our disproportionately high intake of Omega 6 in plant oils.

8. PROCESSED FOOD – WHY IT IS BEST AVOIDED
(We All Know But Let's Spell It Out)

- **Refined Foods:** Such as bread made from refined white flour will have all its nutrients stripped in the processing. Synthetic vitamins reintroduced at a later stage will not function and be bioavailable to the body in the same way as natural wholefoods can offer.

- **Refined Carbohydrates:** Have crept into our diet in such quantities, they are generally low fibre foods and lead to constant blood sugar surges, insulin resistance, diabetes and feed the bad bacteria in our gut.

- **Sugar and High Fructose Corn Syrup:** It is inescapable. Western society adds sugar to tea, coffee, canned drinks, fruit juice, squashes, puts it in cereal … puts it on top of cereal … adds it to yoghurts and savoury food and savoury sauces not to mention the oceans of biscuits, cakes, breads, sweets, chocolate etc, etc … Adding sugar to processed food increases its shelf life.

- **Processed Foods are Made to Press All Your Buttons:** Leaving you wanting more and more and more. The food manufacturer's aim is to produce "hyper-rewarding" products that leave you totally addicted.

- **Heating:** Most processed foods undergo heat treatment that generally destroys heat sensitive vitamins and damages unstable cooking oils.

- **Vegetable Oil:** is used in most processed foods as it is much cheaper than animal fat but it is high in Omega 6 and our over consumption of it leads to chronic inflammation when not balanced with Omega 3. The heated polyunsaturated fat of vegetable oils can lead to inflammation and disease.

- **Additives, Preservatives, Flavourings, Colour, Texture Enhancing Chemicals:**
- The more chemicals are added to a food the harder your body will have to work in order for it to metabolise and get rid of those chemicals. These foods do not add value but use up nutrients in your body that could be used to enhance and protect you instead.

- **Low in Fibre:** A common characteristic of most chemically processed food is that it is low in fibre.

- **Deodorising:** Due to the processing of food some items will actually go rancid and the resulting unpleasant smells need to be disguised through deodorising techniques. An example of this can occur in the processing of vegetable oils.(23)

- **Quality:** Due to the very nature of processing the initial whole foods selected to be included in the final processed article is unrecognisable and the quality can be compromised. For example foods containing processed meats.

- **Storage and Transit:** From the moment fresh food is picked it starts to lose many of its beneficial nutrients. The longer the food spends in transit and storage the less benefit it is likely to offer you.

9. IGNORING THE MICROBIOME

Our Fear Of Bugs Could Be Killing Us (24)

Do you know who you really are?
Healthy humans have around 100, 000,000,000,000 (that's 100 trillion microbes) in their gut.

The gut alone contains 10 times more of these microbes than human cells in the rest of our body put together.

So it can be said that 90% of what we are is effectively a constantly evolving and changing mass of bugs! Known as our microbiome, microbiota, microflora, gut flora, gut bacteria or simply bugs in our gut.

That thought on its own is as empowering as it is frightening…..

Empowering because if you get sick then you really do have a chance through good food and good choices to get well again. Wholesome, nutrient dense food has enormous beneficial power on the bugs in your gut. Frightening because all the bad habits and toxic lifestyles we pursue also have very fundamental and negative impacts on us. Our bugs are constantly evolving and responding to our food and lifestyle choices including stress and sleep.

Our obsession with cleanliness and the use of antibacterial wipes and sprays means that our immediate environment is more sterile than, it now appears, it ought to be. These habits and others that we pursue to eradicate bacteria around us could be causing us much more serious problems than we realised. We are predominantly a mass of bugs and it is apparently very important for us to be much more interconnected with the bugs in the outside world that bring us healthy microbial diversity. If we feed ourselves properly we strengthen the many good microbial communities in our gut that protect us from the rogue pathogens.

How Should Your Microbes Work For You

I say 'should' because many of us are actively doing things that weaken our microbiota or 'gut flora' and in turn weakening ourselves (that I will highlight later).

Our gut flora should work to give us:
- Our protective immune system (around 75% of it is controlled by our gut flora).
- Protection from infection
- Healthy regulation of our metabolism
- Good digestive health
- Vitamins and compounds created by our gut flora for healthy body function
- Mental clarity and good brain function.
- Help reduce our potential for inflammation by protecting us from the damage we inflict through our poor lifestyle choices

   A neglected microbiota can eventually wreak havoc on our bodies.

Microbes Rule

The greater the variety of good bugs you have in your gut the healthier you are likely to be

Although there have been pockets of understanding throughout the ages of this topic, it has largely gone ignored and misunderstood in recent history. It can even be said that such things as pasteurization, refrigeration, disinfectants and antibiotics have not served us as well as we may have thought. These features have put a barrier between us and the microbial world. It is becoming apparent, instead, that the more access we have to the vast array of bugs around us the more diversity of bugs we build up in our gut. That, it now transpires, is the secret of good health.

Our Well Intentioned Actions Have Been Disrupting This Amazing System That Has Taken All of History to Evolve

The use of Antibiotics is just one example of how we have been inadvertently altering this delicate microbiotic system. For antibiotics act indiscriminately going in to kill the good bugs that we rely on for good health as well as the bad bugs.

So although antibiotics have protected, for example, millions of children from dying from infectious diseases over the past 70 years, in the long term the use of antibiotics may be contributing to a fundamental change to the effectiveness and strength of our microbiota. This diminishing strength has translated as a diminished strength in our collective immune systems that has lead to the advent of an ever more common feature of modern illness – Autoimmune Disease. (25)

Listing Auto Immune Disorders Gives a Snap Shot of our Modern World:

- Type 1 Diabetes
- Allergies
- Lupus
- Autism
- Sjogren's Syndrome
- Fibromyalgia
- Colitis
- Crohns Disease
- Chronic Fatigue Syndrome

- Rheumatoid Arthritis
- Coeliac Disease
- Aspergers
- Multiple Sclerosis
- Graves Disease
- Psoriasis
- Hashimoto's Thyroditis
- Inflammatory Bowel Disease

Autism and The Gut/Brain Axis

There is rapidly developing interest in the gut/brain axis as the conditions along the autism spectrum appear to be increasing. (26) Here too it seems that it is often the case that whilst a lot of attention is given to coping with the symptoms of autism with management techniques, not enough, if any, attention is given to the possible gut dysbiosis (microbial imbalance) that may exist and be causing or worsening the condition in individuals with autism. In this area the neurologist and nutritionist Dr Natasha Campbell McBride wrote a comprehensive account of her learning experience in helping her own autistic son, the nutritional protocol she developed and the clinical experiences she gained with patients she went on to treat. Her work was published in 2010 in the book "Gut and Psychology Syndrome – Natural Treatment for Autism, Dyspraxia, ADD, ADHD, Dyslexia, Depression and Schizophrenia".

What Is Weakening Our Immunity?

Things That Are Said to Be Weakening Our Gut Flora/Immune System

- Antibiotics   - Disinfectant sprays   - Caesarian births   - Steroids
- The Pill   - Pollution   - Chemicals & toxins   - Pharmaceuticals
- Anti acids   - Antibacterial gels   - Processed foods
- Sugar ....as this will feed the pathogens/bad bugs that go toward tipping the balance of good bugs to bad in your gut.

Even immensely beneficial aspects like clean water, sanitation and the pasturisation of milk although life-saving, have also impacted in the long term to leave us less robust and open to new autoimmune conditions that were less prevalent before. I think the expression is we have borrowed from Peter to pay Paul .....

Weakening of Our Immune Systems Down Our More Recent Generations

After a number of generations these recent social changes and habits have slowly altered and reduced the number of beneficial microbes that our grandmothers were able to pass on, through breast feeding and natural childbirth, to our mothers who in turn passed on to us and we then passed onto our children. With each generation the gut bacteria became slightly weaker than before.

So it is that today many more children seem to be born with allergies and develop asthma, autism and many other conditions that may not simply be being diagnosed due to 'better diagnosis techniques' but possibly because of ever weakening

immune systems due to diminished gut flora being passed down the generations.
In 2005 an estimated 5,658,900 people had been diagnosed with Asthma (approximately 1 in 9 of the population). Approximately 32,577,300 prescriptions were issued for the condition in 2005 alone. (27) In 1927 when the Asthma Research Council, now known as Asthma UK was founded there were estimated to be around 200,000 cases of asthma in the UK.

Spotlight on Caesarian Sections

One of the most fundamental ways that our microbes (and inherent immune system) pass down the generations is through the birthing process. The microbes that a baby ingests and it's skin is covered in during its exit through the birth canal are invaluable. Notably the lactobacilli flourishes in the mother's vagina during pregnancy and makes the birth canal more acidic giving powerful protection against the more alkali-loving pathogens.

A mother's water's breaking is a far more significant event than most of us appreciate. As the waters splash onto the mother's thighs it spreads the bacteria that the waters have swept up as it came through the vagina. The Lactobacilli is transported onto the mother's skin and colonises her entire skin surface extremely quickly. By the time the baby makes contact with it's mother's skin and suckles on her nipples nature has not only ensured a safe, pathogen free environment for the newborn but also that the baby incorporates this age-old and vital microbe into its own immune system.

Caesarian sections can be life saving for both the mother and child in some cases but today we see it, perhaps, being offered too easily, without mothers understanding the true costs.

By not passing through the birth canal, a baby born by C-section may not be starting life with the same advantages of a baby born naturally. In addition due to surgery it is probable that the mother receives antibiotics in the process adding to the impact of microbial loss.

All is not lost for those children who are born by C section as good diet and the right foods can go a long way to address the disadvantage. Yet disadvantage it may well scientifically turn out to be and these children may be more prone to allergies, asthma, ear infections as they grow. (28)

In more enlightened hospitals techniques are becoming available to minimise this microbial loss to babies born by C-section.

How Can We Strengthen Our Gut Flora And Then Our Immune System

List of Things That Could Benefit Our Gut Flora

- **Owning a dog!**

- **Gardening**

- **Opening the windows** … and letting fresh air and a fresh exchange of bugs into our highly insulated, double glazed homes and offices.

- **Probiotics** can help to increase the number of good bacteria in your gut. Sources: fermented food eg yogurt, sauerkraut, cheese. Homemade fermented food can provide much more potent forms of probiotics than the probiotic capsules available over the counter.

- **Prebioticsie Fibre** on the other hand there are food sources that do not add bacteria directly but rather serve to feed existing bacteria in the gut and strengthen your immune system. Sources: Soluble and Insoluble Fibre found in oats, beans, vegetables and other plant based foods. Our bugs benefit from feeding off the fibre and the polyphenol phytonutrients that are bound to the fibre.

- **Polyphenol Phytonutrients** there are more than 4,000 of these compounds that we know of to date found in plant foods. Very many of them are antioxidants that counteract the damaging effects of free radicals in our body. They can protect against inflammation and reduce tumour growth. They are responsible for the strong flavours and bright colours in plant foods and help defend plants from insect attack.

Examples:
Allicin in garlic, onions, leeks   *Resveratrol in red wine*
Quercetin in citrus fruits, apples, onions   *Curcumin in turmeric*
Capsaicin in chilli and paprika
Rosmarinic acid in rosemary, sage, thyme, peppermint and oregano

The Most Significant Contribution to Gut Health is Believed to be Fibre from Whole Plant Foods and Polyphenols [29]

Fibre and polyphenols are "bioactive food components" that interact with our gut flora and provide them with their main energy source. High whole plant food diets increase our well being by *"up-regulating our beneficial commensal bacteria .* You heard it here first – the jargon of the future ... in other words increasing our gut bacteria's ability to positively respond and interact with its surroundings and keep us functioning well. (See page Spotlight on Polyphenol Phytonutrients)

Faecal transplants .... Don't recoil in horror, this process is generating more and more interest. It has been used to successfully treat people in hospital. More people today after an operation have even further weakened immunity and are more likely to develop an infection known as C Difficile. This infection has had a lot of coverage in the media. It is a notoriously difficult and dangerous pathogen to treat that has been developing resistance to antibiotics. But patients who have been treated through the use of faecal transplants for this infection have nearly all been cured (96%). The transplant will come from a donor who has a healthy profile of bugs living in their intestine that can fight off C Difficile. [30] (Next time you hear the expression 'brown gold' you will know what they are talking about!)

Obesity - Antibiotics and Why You Need to Eat Your Greens

There is a growing school of thought that there is a link between obesity and our individual make up of microbes in our gut. Two main aspects to shed light on are:

Antibiotics

Farmers have known for over 50 years that giving farm animals such as cattle low dose antibiotics increases their weight and therefore their value in meat weight. The antibiotics change the structure of the microbiota in the host that can lead to a metabolic, immune and hormonal imbalance that leads to weight gain. Our consumption of these foods together with our own personal cases of antibiotic intake, especially in childhood may be another factor that has contributed towards the obesity epidemic in modern society.

Firmicutes and Bacteriodetes

Although we can have thousands of different types of bacteria in and on our bodies there are two main 'family' groups that these diverse bacteria come under – Firmicutes and Bacteriodetes. If you have not heard these two words yet you will … a lot! There are about 50 phyla or 'family groups' of bacteria that we know of in the world today. Of the fifty 'phyla', six of these make up 99.9% of all the bacteria in and on your body and these include the two largest groups, Firmicutes and the Bacteriodetes.

A landmark study by Harvard University wanted to analyse the difference in microbial characteristics of 15 healthy children in the European Union and 14 healthy children in a rural African village called Burkina Faso. The study has become so famous that it is often just referred to as the Burkina Faso study. What the study showed was that the African children had a much higher ratio of Bacteriodetes compared to Firmicutes and the European children were the other way round with a much higher ratio of Firmicutes.

Importantly the Bacteriodetes in the African community were able to maximise their energy intake from fibre and were protected from inflammation and intestinal diseases. Their diet was low in fat and animal protein and rich in fibre, starch and vegetables. They were on average breast-fed until the age of two compared to one year in the European children. From then onwards the European children's diet was rich in fat, protein and sugar and low in fibre particularly resistant starches. This diet is associated with a rapid increase in intestinal diseases. (31)

Altering Your Ratio

In the Harvard study they stated that 'it was reasonable to surmise that an increase in the Firmicutes to Bacteriodetes ratio in European children, probably driven by ....diet, might predispose them to future obesity. This F/B ratio may also be considered a useful obesity biomarker. '

With high levels of Firmicutes seemingly not being desirable, to the point that they can alter the behaviour of our genes and trigger inflammation, diabetes, poor heart health as well as obesity, it is perhaps a relief to know that by slowly but significantly increasing the amount of fibre in our diet with plant based food we can quite rapidly improve our F/B ratio. (32)

The Microbiome is Even More ....

We have been lead to believe that our genes come from the sperm and egg of our parents. It would appear that in reality about 23,000 genes come from our parents but the bacteria in our gut is thought to account for around 3 million more genes!(33) This is one of the reasons why the study of Epigenetics is showing us that we have far more control than we previously thought over our health. Our lifestyle and dietary choices have significant influence over whether or not we trigger our genes and become ill or remain healthy.

A very good article introducing the Microbiome to readers in The Economist magazine of August 18, 2012 wrote:

> *".... Evolution has aligned the interests of host and bugs.*
> *In exchange for raw materials and shelter the microbes that*
> *live in and on people feed and protect their hosts, and are thus*
> *integral to that host's well being. Neither wishes the other harm."*

Time to Rethink Our "War" on Bugs

Science is swinging round today, in a quite dramatic way, back to the importance of the Microbiome, gut health and our whole approach to our 'war' on bugs.

Caution and Balance and a New Type of Medicine

When it comes to the microbiome the phrase 'one size fits all' certainly does not apply. The microbiome shows us just how different we are to each other and a reason why we all react differently to our environment, foods and medication.

As our knowledge of the microbiome evolves there is also more understanding that the so called 'bad bugs' (pathogens) are not necessarily out and out 'bad'. Take the pathogen H Pylori – it is well known to the medical community. The general approach to date is that if you have it in your gut it is best treated to remove it. However recent studies have shown that in fact H Pylori may be a good thing to have in youth as it may help protect children against asthma. In fact research conducted through statistical analysis showed that individuals with H Pylori were 40% less likely to develop asthma.

Therefore another contributing factor for the increased incidence of asthma today may be due to the fact that with better sanitation and hygiene in general, it is less likely that this age old pathogen, which has been passed down the generations, is not as prevalent amongst humans as it once was.

In older people however H Pylori can go on to produce problems such as reflux, ulcers and stomach cancer.

Perhaps the case of H Pylori throws up, in fact, a good example of how medicine may evolve in the future as we become more knowledgeable in the field of gut bacteria. Doctors may be able to add or remove strains of bacteria in order to prevent or cure individual conditions. (34)

CHAPTER THREE
ENDING THE GLOOM EMPOWERED BY
EVOLVING AND TRADITIONAL KNOWLEDGE

1. FIBRE, FIBRE, FIBRE

- Western diet does not easily offer enough fibre.
- If we focused on just two things – reduce our sugar intake and increase our fibre intake we would all be a lot better off.
- Fibre comes from plant foods.
- It is important to have both insoluble and soluble fibre.
- A high fibre diet will slow down digestion and especially slow down the absorption of sugars, protecting the liver from being overwhelmed, avoiding spikes in blood sugars, reducing insulin and thus protecting against diabetes.
- Fibre also helps the liver to eliminate toxins and excess fat from the body faster. Fibre gives a feeling of fullness and helps in weight loss.
- Increasing fibre into the diet is very important but needs to be done slowly to avoid bloating, cramps and constipation or diarrhoea and water should be consumed in reasonable quantity to keep everything working efficiently.

Insoluble fibre
It helps promote regularity and healthy digestion. It does not dissolve in water and creates 'bulk' in the digestive tract enabling it to 'sweep' through the bowels keeping them clear and reducing the risk of constipation, haemorrhoids and colon cancer. If loose stools are a problem the bulk-forming insoluble fibre helps to absorb water and solidify waste.

Sources:
The pulp and the peel of berries and many fruits, legumes, the skins and pulp of vegetables, nuts and seeds are all good sources. Do not be tempted to stick to one source just because it has a higher fibre content than others. It is important to alternate and keep your diet diverse.

Soluble fibre
It helps stabilise blood sugar levels it manages diarrhoea and some symptoms of an irritable bowel. It protects against intestinal ulcers and feeds the good bacteria in your gut helping them to flourish over pathogens.

Sources:
Again we are looking at legumes, oatmeal (also high in iron, magnesium, phosphorus and potassium). Most vegetables have a high fibre content, cruciferous vegetables particularly Brussels sprouts are high in soluble fibre. Fruit also, is good for both types of fibre, such as citrus fruits, apricots and mangoes. Flaxseed is a good source of soluble fibre. If you pour water over flaxseed you can easily see the jelly like consistency that develops that is so effective for the gut.

Remember to incorporate raw food as well – salads are a good vessel for this – we can be imaginative and diverse in our choice of ingredients: spring onions, avocado, red cabbage, bell peppers, beetroot, radishes, sugar snap peas, carrots, different salads, nuts, seeds, celery, herbs, fennel bulbs, the list of raw foods for our salads goes on. Also lightly steamed vegetables such as asparagus, mange tout, etc, etc. Many of these foods will contain both the soluble and insoluble fibre that we need and remember to chew slowly!

When we eat good quantities of fibre through vegetables for example, the fibre and antioxidants can help counteract an occasional indiscretion of something sweet when consumed within a meal.

Fibre and Cholesterol

If the liver feels there is a surplus of cholesterol to requirements it expels it via the intestine. Our bodies should be consuming more fibre than we do today in order to quickly and efficiently push out the excess cholesterol (our ancestors were consuming as much as ten times more fibre than we do). Instead we are not clearing our system as quickly and cholesterol together with other compounds may linger and be reabsorbed via the intestinal wall. Increasing our fibre intake will help clear our system of the cholesterol that the liver no longer wants.

We Have To Face It In The End – We Need To Eat Our Greens

I know I am stating the obvious but let us remind ourselves why. There is no escaping the fact that eating a diverse and good amount of vegetables daily is a one of the best things we can do for our health.

Vegetables and other plant-based foods provide pre-biotics, fibre, vitamins, minerals, and phytonutrients. Importantly also, they feed our good bugs and allow them to flourish. When it comes to our microbes, diversity is key. Focusing repeatedly on the same foods can lead to some bacteria in your gut, although healthy, to flourish too much and become more dominant than they should, leading to imbalance which is never ideal.

Vegetables and plant based foods, thanks to their fibre content make us feel full, assist our digestive health and provide us with a richness of nutrients, providing we buy carefully and eat them together with some fat to enable us to absorb the fat soluble vitamins they contain. Put butter on warm vegetables and good quality olive oil on salads or cold vegetable dishes.

There are so many fantastic recipe dishes to discover to enable us to thoroughly enjoy eating our vegetables. Recipes that include adding eggs, herbs and spices.

I believe vegetables should be the main part of our plate with a condiment of olive oil or butter together with a small side portion of meat or fish. Meat and fish are some of the richest food sources of vitamins and minerals but should be eaten in moderation. We want to leave plenty of room for the true stars that provide the fibre, phytonutrients and prebiotic benefits for our gut.

2. FEEDING FOODS & REPAIRING FOODS

Why We Need our Fruit and Vegetables but Also our Meat and Fish

Protein Promotes Cell Duplication

Protein and in particular animal protein can be categorised as a feeding food. It spurs on the duplication of cells and is important to be consumed when in the growing or the reproductive phase of life.

When it comes to the amount of essential nutrients in food and increasing our chances of consuming healthy levels of these essential vitamins and minerals we can, if we are not careful, put ourselves at a severe disadvantage if we stick only to plant based foods. Animal produce provides much more concentrated doses of nutrients that help feed and strengthen our bodies. Some essential vitamins are only available in animal foods such as Vitamin B12 and the Retinoid form of Vitamin A.

However, according to new research carried out at the University of Southern California by, amongst others, Biogerontologist, Dr Valter Longo, excessive animal protein consumption, including milk and cheese is associated with a dramatic rise in cancer in the middle aged, compared to those who consumed low quantities of animal protein.

Protein Intake and Lifespan

Longo's research focused on the hormone Insulin-like Growth Factor-1(IGF-1). Moderate to high consumption of animal protein increased the level of this hormone. Although necessary for proper growth in children, the study revealed it contributed significantly to the growth of tumours in middle aged individuals.

The study, looked at the dietary intake of over 83,000 people in the US over 18 years. IGF-1, according to the study, although enabling our body to grow when young, makes us more vulnerable to cancer in mid life. Then IGF-1 levels tail off after the age of 65 leading to frailty and loss of muscle. According to Longo, animal protein consumption would need to be re-considered at higher levels once again, in old age, in order to stay a healthy weight and be more protected from disease.

Because of the emphasis placed for many years on high protein consumption due to the Atkins diet and the Paleolithic diet, researchers may have reduced the focus on the adverse effects of high meat consumption. Longo's study showed that even people who ate a moderate (up to 20% of total calories) amount of animal protein were three times at greater risk of cancer than those on a low protein diet (less than 10% of total calories). (35)

(Longo's research on the IGF-1 hormone, longevity and fasting was in part a catalyst to the 5:2 diet popularized by Dr Michael Mosely following his meeting with Valter Longo during the making of the BBC2 Horizon documentary "Eat, Fast & Live Longer" in 2012).

Plant Based Food and Cell Repair

Fruit and vegetables are essential in a healthy diet. Apart from the good amount of fibre they provide, together with essential vitamins and minerals they also provide very many precious and varied phytonutrients. These are compounds that are not available in animal based foods and provide the body with a massive range of cell repairing tools.(36)

Spotlight on Polyphenol Phytonutrients and the Benefits of Plant Foods (37)

Scientists are continuing to identify unique, plant-based phytonutrients. The phytonutrient message is aim for colour variety.

Plant based foods contain over 4,000 groups of different polyphenol phytonutrients. These compounds are responsible for, amongst other things, the

68

bright colour and strong tastes of plant foods. Phytonutrients may well account for the health benefits shown in plant based whole foods in preventing and fighting cancer.

Variety and Availability

Greater variety of plant foods enhances health benefits. Polyphenol phytonutrients in plants add to the healthy mix providing us with many types of valuable anti-oxidants. Their richest sources are sometimes in the skin of the plant so peeling can remove all or most of the health benefit. Polyphenol content may be highest at the food's freshest time and cooking can also reduce the benefits to us of these compounds.

Target Colour

Phytonutrients have been divided into five colours: Green, Red, White, Purple/Blue and Yellow/Orange. A basic goal should therefore be to eat 2 of each colour a day.

Red Foods

For Heart, Dna, Prostate And Urinary Tract Health
Well known example: **Lycopene**   Source: Cooked Tomatoes

Orange/Yellow Foods

For Eye And Immune Health, Supporting Growth And Development
Well known examples:
Alpha-carotene Source: pumpkin, carrots for cardiovascular health
Beta-carotene Source: peppers – cos or romaine lettuce, kale.

Purple/Blue Foods

For Brain And Cognitive Health And Heart, Arteries, Bone.   Protects Against
Cancers And Aging Effects.
Well known example:
Resveratrol Source: Red wine

Green Foods

For Eye And Gum Health, Lung, Liver, Arterial And Cell Function. Protects Against
Cancers
Well known example:
Lutein/Zeaxanthin Source: Kale – Spinach- Paprika

White Foods

For Bone, Circulatory And Heart Health And Arterial Function.   Protects Against
Cancer.
Well Known example:
Allicin Source: Garlic – onions – leeks
Quercetin Source: onions – citrus fruits – apples

When searching for the richest beneficial sources of polyphenols in plant foods the
results can vary depending on what test methods are used (eg Folin, ORAC, or
FRAP). Consideration needs to be given to the bioavailability of these compounds
ie how easily we can absorb them and the quantity of food that we actually
consume of their sources.   For example dried herbs and spices are very
concentrated sources but we only consume them in small quantities anyway.

That said, however, it appears that there is a number of repeatedly present
categories of food that show up at the top of most lists no matter who is measuring
the levels of polyphenols: herbs (especially dried) and spices, tea (green and
black), cocoa and red wine, fruits include berries and apples (skin), vegetables

include globe artichokes, red onions, red chicory, spinach, broccoli and endives, nuts and seeds, olives and extra virgin olive oil.

Whatever we read, however, we must always remember that "variety is the spice of life" especially for our friendly bugs!

Top Tip To Make You Tip Top

Garlic but specifically Allicin in garlic can act as an effective, natural antibiotic but it also has certain anti-viral and anti-fungal and anti-cancer properties.

Allicin has been shown to prevent blood clotting by 89-90%, in a study it was a "significantly more potent platelet inhibitor than aspirin at nearly equivalent concentrations."[38] Although it is not rich in vitamins and minerals it has a wealth of healing traits that has made it valuable and sought after throughout history.

TOP TIP – Allicin is the crucial health-giving enzyme and it is only formed when the garlic is crushed and alliin and alliinase enzymes merge to produce allicin. In addition to this, one must wait a few minutes before heating the garlic otherwise the heat sensitive allinase is destroyed before it can create the allicin and you risk missing all its benefits. So when we start cooking we should always crush our garlic first and set it aside for 10 minutes to work its magic.

Get Excited About Herbs And Spices (39)

We can tell by their flavour that they pack an extra big punch. We should use every opportunity to incorporate and combine them into our cooking, whether it is soups, salads, vegetable or meat or fish dishes.

The goodness of herbs and spices is highly concentrated and alternating and maintaining variety is important. Incorporating these regularly into our cooking is a great thing to do.

Let's remind ourselves of some of them, some of the most powerful are:

Spices	Curcumin/Turmeric	Ginger	Coriander seeds
Star Anise	Fennel Seeds	Chilli	Carraway
Capers	Saffron	Cardamon	Black Pepper
Curry Powder	Cayenne Pepper	Paprika	Cloves
Cinnamon	Nutmeg	Cumin	
Herbs	Basil	Parsley	Dill
Fennel	Marjoram	Rosemary,	Coriander
Sage	Thyme	Tarragon	Oregano
Peppermint			

Not to mention all the wonderful aromatic flavours in Thai and south east Asian cooking .....

Like everything else – it is good to alternate the herbs and spices we use and be generous when cooking with them!.

.... And What About Nuts?

Maastricht University in the Netherlands published a study in June 2015 carried out within an observational study, running since 1986, of 120,000 Dutch men and women between the ages of 55-69 years old. (40)

Nut consumption was assessed, taking into account portion size and frequency.

Nut and peanut consumption lowered the risk of death from several major diseases over those who did not eat nuts. The strongest reductions in mortality appeared in respiratory and neurodegenerative disease and diabetes, followed by cancer and cardiovascular disease.

The project leader Professor Piet van den Brandt (Epidemiologist) observed of the results: "it was remarkable that substantially lower mortality was already observed at consumption levels of 15 grams of nuts or peanuts on average per day (less than a handful). A higher intake was not associated with further reduction in mortality risk."

Nuts are rich in vitamins, fibre, antioxidants and other bioactive polyphenols. They also contain monounsaturated fats and polyunsaturated fats (enough Omega 6 can be consumed from moderate nut consumption and Omega 6 should be kept to a minimum in additional sources). Peanut butter, also included in the study, did not show improvement in mortality rates. Raising the point that peanut butter also contains processed vegetable oils.

I am wary of nut flours such as almond flour as it may be too concentrated and too easy to over consume almonds (a cup of almond flour can contain approximately 90 almonds).

Nuts are another good example of why moderation and diversity is always important. As the above study shows, there is little further benefit noted in consuming more than half a handful of nuts a day and more may lead to over consumption of pro-inflammatory Omega 6 and other negative consequences.

The Super Powers Of Traditional Stocks And Broths

Chicken Stock And Bone Broth

So Much Incredible Goodness, So Cheap and So Easy
Today we tend to buy much of our meat filleted. The routine of making stock out of left over bone and cartilage once common, is now rare.

"We're missing a trick if you are not making stocks and broths" Whether a child, a young adult rushing around, an elderly person or someone suffering from ill health, homemade stocks and broths offer an incredible source of important goodness in an easy to digest way.

Easy to make - versatile to consume - full of goodness
Easy to digest – amazing value compared to supplements

What Makes a Good Stock or Broth?

A good broth or stock is an opportunity to incorporate into our diets nutrients and proteins that are often missed opportunities, wastefully discarded in modern diets that can be obtained through the skin, cartilage and bone of animals and that offer health and vitality in a versatile and nutrient dense way. Many of the nutrients on offer in stocks and broths are being purchased at great expense in nutritional supplements.

Even if you don't follow the recipes included here to the letter and you cut corners – the important thing is that you incorporate stocks into your routine. Add them to soups, gravy or absorb it into rice.

Stocks are a big nutritional leap forward for all the family.

.... So Why Are They So Great?

74

What Do Stocks And Broths Contain That Are So Good For You?

Calcium, Magnesium, Phosphorous, Potassium, Silicon, Sulphur, Trace Minerals (All sold as expensive supplements).For children and the elderly bone stock offers good levels of both highly absorbable calcium and magnesium to promote bone and dental health amongst other things.

Sulphur Attracts toxic compounds and draws them out of the body. (NB other sulphur containing foods that do this are garlics, onions and cruciferous vegetables.

Cysteine that forms Glutathione (Sold as an expensive supplement) Aids the breakdown of mucous in the lungs, a very powerful antioxidant and an important detoxifier that assists in drawing out heavy metals from the body such as cadmium, lead and mercury. Transports nutrients for immune system function

Glycine: (Sold as an expensive supplement). Is found in significantly greater concentrations in skin and bones of animals than in meat. Glycine helps fight inflammation. It has significant effect on mental health, is calming and aids good sleep.

Glucosamine: (Sold as an expensive supplement). Although produced in the body, as we grow older levels can diminish. Stocks and broths offer it and help to maintain healthy joints and cartilage and counteract age related arthritic pain.

Gelatin: An important characteristic of gelatin is that it draws water towards it, so when used in cooking whether a soup with vegetables or a sauce over meat it enables proper and healthy digestion to occur.
Supports healthy hair and nails.

Healing Leaky Gut A good, 'gloopy' gelatin is formed when stock is slow-cooked for a good few hours. For many who suffer from 'Leaky Gut' it helps to heal the lining of the intestines providing easy to digest nutrients. This allows the gut a chance to repair itself and stop larger molecules of food crossing the gut wall. This can be the cause of many allergies and immune disorders.

It offers relief also to serious intestinal disorders such as Crohn's disease, Colitis. Those suffering these conditions would generally find meat difficult to digest, the gelatin in stocks and broths offer easily digestible protein.

Stock Recipes

Chicken Stock Recipe
As ever try to ensure the source of your chicken is the best you can get.
The easiest option is to use the left over carcass of Sunday roast chicken.
Alternatively your butcher may be able to provide you with chicken carcasses if he prepares his own fillets in his shop.
Chicken wings and drumsticks are another option.
The important thing is to include skin, bone and cartilage of the chicken.
Put into a large pot with lid together with:
- 5 litres of water
- 2 tablespoons of vinegar or lemon (this helps to draw out the minerals)
- 1 large onion coarsely chopped
- 2 large carrots coarsely chopped
- 3 celery sticks coarsely chopped
- A handful of unchopped parsley
- Some Bay Leaves
- Sprinkle of Peppercorns

Instructions
- Place your carcass and chicken pieces in pot with the water and vinegar this will begin the leaching process of minerals from the bones.
- Add the vegetables.
- Add the water and vinegar and let stand for an hour.
- Bring to the boil but do not allow to boil too long. This will bring scum to the surface that can then be skimmed off.
- Add herbs and spices you wish to include and leave to simmer with lid on.

- Cook on hob at lowest temperature that allows a very gentle simmer to occur or in the oven if you prefer, at just over 110 degrees ensuring that a gentle simmer is occurring.
- Cook for a minimum of 6 hours and up to 24 hours. The longer, the better the flavour.
- You will not experience the 'gloop' until the stock has been allowed to cool.
- It is best not to leave stocks hanging around at room temperature for too long as this ideal temperature for bugs to breed.
- Once the stock has been removed from heat. Allow to cool slightly and then place pot in a sink half filled with cold water. This will allow the pot to cool slightly faster.
- Strain the stock in a colander removing all meat, bones, vegetables and herbs.
- Once cooled either:
1. Place pot in fridge over night and in the morning you will find that the stock has congealed and formed a layer of fat on top. Skim off the fat. The stock below will be a lovely jelly consistency ready to be divided into containers or ice cube trays and placed in the freezer for storage.
2. Stir fat back in and divide into containers.

You can store for several days in the fridge and several months in the freezer.

Bone Stock Recipe

As before try to obtain the best quality source of food that you can.
Variety is important for a healthy bone stock so ask the butcher what he can offer you. Some butcher's prepare bone bags for consumption by pets. Chopped bones where the marrow is exposed is great as it provides a lot of nutrients and flavour. Also include pieces of meat on the bone like rib or neck.
- 1.5 kg of bone with marrow and1 kg of meat on bone eg ribs or neck
- 2 tablespoons of vinegar (this helps to draw out the minerals)
- 1 large onion, 2 large carrots, 3 celery sticks coarsely chopped
  To be added after skimming off of surface scum has occurred:

- A handful of unchopped parsley (some leave this for only the last 10 minutes of cooking time)
- Some Bay Leaves
- Other sprigs of herbs of choice, tied for easy removal later
- Sprinkle of Peppercorns

Instructions

- Place your bones with marrow in pot with the water and vinegar this will begin the leaching process of minerals from the bones.
- Meanwhile roast the bones with meat on them until brown.
- Add the roasted bones to the pot of bones in water and add the vegetables.
- Ensure water level is up to an inch below rim of pot.
- Bring to the boil but do not allow to boil too long. This will bring scum to the surface that can then be skimmed off.
- Add desired herbs and spices and leave to simmer with lid on.
- Cook on hob at lowest temperature that allows a very gentle simmer to occur or in the oven at just over 110 degrees ensuring that it has reached a very gentle simmer.
- Bone stock should ideally cook for a minimum of 12 hours and up to 72 hours. Though in my experience I have reached a lovely gelatinous gloop after just 8 hours!
- You will not experience the 'gloop' until the stock has been allowed to cool.
- It is best not to leave stocks hanging around at room temperature for too long as this ideal temperature for bugs to breed.
- Once the stock has been removed from heat. Allow to cool slightly and then place pot in a sink half filled with cold water. This will allow the pot to cool slightly faster.
- Strain stock in a colander removing all meat, bones, vegetables and herbs.
- Once cooled place pot in fridge over night.
- In the morning you will find that the stock has congealed and formed a layer of fat. This can be removed and stored in the fridge for use as fat for cooking. The stock below will be a lovely jelly consistency ready to divide into containers or ice cube trays and placed in the freezer for storage.
- Stock can be stored for several days in the fridge and several months in the freezer.

.... And Don't Forget Fish Stock

In Asia and the Mediterranean the tradition of fish stock is more prevalent. Have you met anyone recently trying to persuade their fishmonger to give them the left over fish heads to make a good stock? Fish stock is rich in minerals including iodine and fish heads contain the benefits of the thyroid gland.

Stocks and Broths are Gentle on the Gut and Nurture You Well When You are Unwell

Stocks and broths are gentle on the digestive system. They are good nutritious ways of taking in more goodness when feeling unwell and off your food. They are especially good for those suffering from digestive and inflammatory issues as they allow the gut to heal but still feed the body.

3. REPAIR YOUR GUT AND STRENGTHEN IMMUNITY

Probiotics foods Supply your intestine with trillions of beneficial bacteria, especially from fermented foods.

Prebiotic foods Supply the beneficial bacteria already living in your intestine with the plant foods it needs to thrive

Probiotic Food and The Forgotten Art of Fermentation

Before refrigeration was invented fermentation was the method used for thousands of years, by people all over the world, to preserve and store food for months/years. Examples of these foods range from alcohol, cheese, sauerkraut, yoghurt, kefir, kimchi and many, many more, as just about anything can be fermented.

Fermented food is an extremely valuable but lost art in western society. It provides the body with huge amounts of beneficial good bacteria for a healthy digestive system leading to a strong immune system. To give you an idea of the strength and value of say, a good, homemade sauerkraut, a teaspoon can provide you with millions more beneficial bacteria than a whole packet of probiotic tablets

War
There is an on-going war between the good bacteria in your gut that keeps you healthy, strong and mentally agile and the bad bugs (pathogens) that live there too. Pathogens thrive on sugar and other refined carbohydrates whilst probiotic fermented foods have the ability to radically increase the population of good bugs thus driving out the pathogens from your gut.(41)

In recent years with the emphasis on bacteria being viewed as simply dangerous, something to be eliminated by antibiotics or antibacterial sprays, the importance of this bacterial balance in the gut has been severely underestimated and even avoided. Fear of bacteria meant that we became unsure of the safety of fermented foods.

We Become Sick When the Pathogens Win the War

In today's sugar-laden society pathogens have the upper hand as we are busy feeding them exactly what they need to thrive. We must take on board once more, as people knew in the past, that in order to have good physical and mental health we must first fix our digestive health.

Sauerkraut and cheeses made from raw milk are my favourite options but there are many options and much written on the subject for you to explore and choose from. I used "The Complete Idiot's Guide to Fermenting Foods" by Wardeh Harmon that set me quickly on a successful and tasty path. In fact my favourite is sauerkraut adding leeks, fennel, fennel seeds and dill to my cabbage as I love the licorice flavour but the guide encourages you to experiment. It also explains why the fermentation process is safe.

Exploding Jars at the Supermarket

With the advent of supermarkets properly fermented vegetables were no longer so viable to sell. Fermentation is an on-going process that produces perfectly safe gaseous by-products but trying to place fermenting sauerkraut on a supermarket shelf would probably result in exploding jars! Fermented vegetables have the same sour, vinegary flavour as modern day pickled vegetables that you do find on the supermarket shelf. These items however are not the product of fermentation but recipes using vinegar itself to provide that same tangy taste to complement meat dishes. Most health benefits are lost though.

Like chicken stocks and bone broth mentioned earlier, this is a food item that is easy to prepare at home and can be made literally by the bucket load and stored in special pickling jars that will last for months and months for the whole family. Remember even just a teaspoon a day is enough to give the immune system a massive boost. I like to eat mine as a condiment with cheese.

Captain Cook and Scurvy

Finally and to press the point home of how marvelous sauerkraut is, it also provides potent anti-inflammatory benefits, it helps to reduce fat (lipids) in the blood stream caused by, for example, the consumption of sugar and is high in Vitamin A and C. In fact sauerkraut can contain up to 200 times more Vitamin C than the original vegetables used to make it.

It was this fact that lead Captain Cook the famous explorer of the 18th century to introduce it as a long term storable foodstuff on board his ships to provide his sailors with Vitamin C through out their epic journeys across the world. He thereby prevented the long-standing problem of scurvy suffered, often fatally, by those embarking on these journeys where fresh food was unobtainable. For this, Captain Cook was awarded the Copley Gold Medal in 1776 by the Royal Society.

Prebiotic Food – Benefits and Sources

Most of us are familiar with Probiotics but not so aware of Prebiotics – a relatively new area of refocus. Prebiotics in the form of plant based fibre serve to feed and increase the number of good bacteria in our gut.

Inulin is an example of a prebiotic that occurs in thousands of plant-based foods. Humans are only able to part digest prebiotics leaving these important, partially digested carbohydrate to provide sustenance to the beneficial bacteria in our gut.

Traditional diets were much richer in prebiotic food and as we are learning more about our microbiota we are learning of the loss to health in not eating these foods. Importantly research has found that many antioxidant rich polyphenols mentioned earlier are often bound to fibre so if we remove the fibre we lose the polyphenol.

Green vegetables and plant foods in general are rich in prebiotics and in particular: onions, garlic, endives, Jerusalem artichokes, asparagus, chicory to name just a few.

Juicing Or Blending?

Juicing and blending have the potential to be very useful ways of enhancing our intake of nutrients in a day and of making it easier to consume our 5, 7 or 10 a day! However, we must be wary of the fructose and keep our blood sugar levels stable.

Blending

For an extra hit of fibre and nutrients in a raw form the blended smoothie is becoming increasingly popular. It is becoming the prevalent opinion that when consuming fruit it is better to go with the blending option not juicing as blending will retain the fibre of the fruit and slow down the absorption of the fructose sugar.

Fresh tasting raw vegetable smoothies are being enjoyed by more and more people. The use of cucumber, celery, mint are cleverly being used to disguise too much of a 'green' flavour and when combined with flavoursome berries, spices and other herbs, the latest smoothie recipes are really worth trying.

Juicing

The advantage that juicing is said to have over blending is that with the fibre removed, the nutrients in the juice have the capacity to be more fully and quickly absorbed through the gut wall. With vegetable juicing this speed and ease of absorption is enhanced and has the potential to act as a fantastic natural supplement/boost of vitamins, minerals and antioxidants.

However, when it comes to fruit, juicing needs to be moderated. Adding apples, pears and other high fructose fruits to your juices will only go to raise your blood sugars too quickly as all the fibre that can go towards tempering that blood sugar high has been removed.

Finally - and a bit of a blow to juicing, we are discovering that the majority of polyphenol phytonutrients may actually be bound to fibre providing further incentive to either eat the whole fruit or vegetable or blend it, to maintain all possible health benefits.(42)

"Swill It Around A While"

Whatever one chooses, juicing or blending, the important thing to remember is that the first stage of digestion occurs in the mouth. When drinking a smoothie or a juice it is important to keep it in the mouth and "swill it around a while" as the enzyme called Amylase that is secreted in the mouth is responsible for the initial digestion of carbohydrate. Allowing smoothies or juices through to our digestive system without being properly digested can cause an array of health issues.

Let's Be Wary of the Fructose Content of the Fruits We Choose to Use

As they contain between 5-10g of fructose per medium portion size, look out for the fructose content of:
   mangoes, grapes, apples, pears, cherries, blueberries and bananas

Fruits such as :
  lime, lemon, cranberries, plums, grapefruit, peaches, raspberries, kiwis, oranges
only contain between 0.2g-3.5g of fructose per medium portion.
(USDA National Nutrient Database).

4. TIME TO PAY MORE ATTENTION TO THE CHEMICAL ASSAULT

"All disease is caused by only two things: deficiency or toxicity."

Toxicity

I heard those words years ago, I do not know who originally said them but they have resonated with me ever since. It led me to paying a bit more attention to products that we buy and use such as cosmetics, domestic cleaning products, fire retardant chemicals and pollution in general that surround us in our modern world. One way or another our bodies' are bombarded with chemicals on a daily basis inhaled and absorbed into our lungs, ingested or absorbed through our skin. Should we be adopting the view that if we are not prepared to eat it then why should we be prepared to put it on our skin!

We should take stock and think whether all these products are really necessary and whether, may be, there are some more natural alternatives we could use instead. It might even work out cheaper. Most of us will have thought along these lines at one time or another but the difference today is that are bodies are in danger of reaching a point of 'saturation'. Marketing machines and mass production have been working flat out and efficiently for decades and the result is that without realising it we have been talked into using so very many products that we didn't even know we needed.

We double glaze our houses, refuse to open our windows and resort to air fresheners ….

5. PARTICULAR VITAMINS & MINERALS TO TAKE A CLOSER LOOK AT

Deficiency

A varied, healthy diet of whole foods that have been thoughtfully sourced for quality and freshness is obviously vital for our health but on my journey I have gone from resisting the idea of supplementation to believing that we have no choice but to supplement if we wish to preserve our well-being. Depending on who we are, what we do and where we live what we need to supplement can vary substantially. Choosing our vitamins and minerals needs to be done carefully and investigated fully, paying attention to our body's ability to absorb what it consumes, the doses we take and the origin of the supplements.

Variation in recommended vitamin supplement dosage is a major subject in itself. For example vitamin C tablets can be found in shops at 500mg when in fact some advocate 6,000mg (discussed later) and upwards a day, spread out over the day. Tablets at 500mg would prove to be a costly way of consuming this high quantity of vitamin C.

I do not believe we can realistically take in all our recommended daily allowance of vitamins and minerals through food alone and in addition, ironically, some of the recommended allowances may be entirely too low.

However there are certain vitamins and minerals that during our evolution over tens of thousands of years may have been more abundant to us such as magnesium (fourth most common element in the earth) and Vitamin D (abundant through sun exposure). We will have evolved to be fundamentally dependent on these easily accessible nutrients. However the lives we led that caused us to evolve in this way do not match the world we live in today. We do not eat the same foods and we do not necessarily get the same amount of time outdoors and thus we can suffer from fundamental deficiencies.

On my journey of discovery I have come across a few vitamins and mineral facts that really stood out. Obviously all the vitamins and minerals, including trace minerals are important to us but the following have been particularly interesting.
Magnesium – Vitamin D – Vitamin K2 – Vitamin C

Magnesium

Magnesium is a vital mineral to our bodies involved in over 300 metabolic functions and essential for maintaining balanced muscle and nerve function.

It is important for healthy bones, steady heart rhythm, stable blood pressure and healthy heart.

If the average person was eating healthily and consuming a plentiful, daily serving of dark leafy greens together with regular consumption of nuts, seeds (particularly pumpkin seeds), dark chocolate, fish and avocados for example, then they would probably be getting sufficient levels of this mineral. Much is said about soil depletion causing lack of magnesium but remember that chlorophyll is what gives a vegetable its green colour and chlorophyll can not form without magnesium.

Reasons For Deficiency

Unfortunately it is believed that many of us do not get enough in our diet. In addition, the sugars and carbohydrates we eat use up our magnesium store as it is needed in significant quantity just simply to metabolise the sugar laden foods we eat.

The situation is the same with chemicals and toxins that enter our body. Here too magnesium is necessary to enable our body to deal with the toxins. For these reasons many of us are severely lacking in this most important mineral to carry out its functions that enable our bodies to work efficiently.

If supplementation is favoured the issue of toxicity is not a problem as excess consumption is regulated by the body and excreted.

Deficiency Can Be Very Serious

One of the signs of deficiency is muscle spasm, a common example is foot or calf cramp typically experienced when in bed especially when stretching but muscle spasm can manifest itself in far more serious ways.

Muscle spasms associated with the arteries and the heart can lead to heart attack and strokes. Sudden death in athletes can be brought on by excess sweating and loss of minerals exacerbated by consumption of sweetened sports drinks that both lead to severe magnesium depletion.

Back Pain

A lot of back pain that is suffered can be attributed to lack of magnesium. The tightening of the very many muscles in our backs from the neck to the lumbago could be addressed with the reduction of sugars and carbohydrates and the replenishing of magnesium levels. Traditional knowledge would have encouraged bathing in Epsom Salts, for their magnesium content and the mineral's absorbability through the skin.

Effect on Other Essential Nutrients

Lack of magnesium will hamper other essential nutrients to carry out their function properly as they require to work in synergy to serve their purposes.

The Magnesium – Calcium Relationship Is Important

Many people, especially women over a certain age are encouraged to supplement their calcium intake but without a proper balance of magnesium it can lead to an increased risk of heart attack, osteoporosis, kidney stones and other issues. . (38)

In simple terms magnesium aids muscle relaxation and calcium aids muscle contraction. When calcium is supplemented and not balanced with magnesium then muscles (including your heart) can be at risk of going into spasm (heart attack).

In addition to this calcium on its own cannot be assimilated into the bone. It needs to work within a team that includes magnesium, Vitamin D and Vitamin K2 (that in turn require other vitamins and minerals to function efficiently). Instead the calcium will remain in the soft tissue causing hardening of tissue through calcification – e.g. hardening of the arteries. (43)

Again these relationships are described in simple terms but highlight just why it is so important to eat well and have a good variety of food to maximise your chances of taking in your vitamins and minerals. It also emphasizes why the need for doctors to understand nutrition is so important.

For further reading on the amazingly vast and important subject of Magnesium I would recommend Dr Carolyn Dean (author of "The Magnesium Miracle") who has been researching the subject for nearly 20 years.

Vitamin C

This vitamin is so important that it is produced in nearly all living organisms both plant and animal. Unfortunately humans lost this ability millions of years ago.

The scientist Irwin Stone said of this event: "….(it) may be eventually regarded as the greatest single physiological and biochemical catastrophe to have happened to Man in the course of evolution"

Vitamin C (also known as ascorbic acid) is a powerful antioxidant. It fights infection and free radicals. It helps us maintain healthy skin, bones, teeth, and blood cells and digestion. It is what keeps us standing as it is vital for the production of collagen that heals our soft tissue and gives it its elasticity.

We are familiar with vitamin C deficiency due to the plight of sailors up until the 1770s who suffered from scurvy on their long sea voyages with no access to the vitamin in their food. Their suffering was characterized by bleeding gums, nose bleeds, rupturing of capillaries and thus bruising and frequent infection.

Today we are told that the RDA (recommended daily allowance) for vitamin C is 90mg. It may be the case though that such a small amount is only enough to prevent the outward signs of scurvy. We may, however, still be significantly deficient in vitamin C to be suffering from the symptoms of scurvy at a sub-clinical level. In other words we may be suffering health problems due to this deficiency but not attributing it to the right cause.

The Question of "Megadosing"

Listening to recordings made by Linus Pauling, a winner of two Nobel Peace Prizes for science and famously the author of "Vitamin C and the Common Cold" I was taken with his explanation of how deficiency of ascorbic acid reduced the elasticity of our arteries and was a major cause for the lesions or small tears in our arteries that can lead us down the path to eventual arterial blockages, strokes and heart attacks.

Linus Pauling advocated taking much higher doses of the vitamin, pointing out that the vast majority of animals produce their own vitamin C and increase this production at moments of stress, injury, illness and trauma. These things together with pollution use up vitamin C and in humans we are left lacking.

Due to a genetic mutation we lost a vital enzyme that animals use to release ascorbic acid in to their bloodstream as and when required.

Unlike other species that also suffered this mutation and died out quickly we survived due to the fact that in jungle areas we had vitamin c-rich food all year round.

According to The Vitamin C Foundation 1997:

"The fact that almost all species continue to make vitamin C suggests that the amount of this vitamin generally available from diet is not enough for optimum nutrition except in exceptional circumstances such as a tropical environment." "…. Under normal circumstances the daily amount produced (in animals), adjusted for comparison to a 70 kg man, is somewhere between 3,000 mg and 15,000 mg, with an average of 5,400 mg."

"More than 50% of people require over 2,500 mg (of ascorbic acid) to reach maximum absorption. "

"Vitamin C is one of the least toxic substances known to man"

Linus Pauling took high levels of Vitamin C staggered throughout the day. He lived to 93 mentally and physically agile.

Vitamin D

There is No Sunshine in the On-Line World

Vitamin D is known as the sunshine vitamin. It is fundamental to health.
Offices, computers, electronic distractions, TV, texting, in other words the 'on-line' world is keeping us indoors and away from the sunshine.

Direct exposure to sunlight is the most efficient way to maximise our vitamin D levels. For those of us not lucky enough to live in the Tropics but in countries where the winters are longer and on top of that those of us that "do not work in the fields" but work indoors, exposure to the sun is fairly limited. In addition to this, today, when we do go outdoors we are encouraged to cover up or wear high protection sunscreen.

Science is busy looking at the whole issue of Vitamin D at the moment and there is an awareness that our fear of exposure to sunlight due to skin cancer needs to be balanced with need for Vitamin D as its deficiency in our bodies is causing many problems.

Vitamin D is fundamentally important for cellular health, helping to prevent certain cancers, including skin cancers![45]. It is required for immunity, bone and muscle function, mood, depression, insomnia, organ and brain health…. Well that's about everything really!

Go Pink But Don't Burn

According to the Vitamin D Council:
"The two main ways to get vitamin D are by exposing your bare skin to sunlight and by taking vitamin D supplements. You can't get the right amount of vitamin D your body needs from food. The most natural way to get vitamin D is by exposing your bare skin to sunlight (ultraviolet B rays)."

92

Depending on who we are, where we live and what we do we are all bound to have very different levels of Vitamin D. It may be the case that testing our Vitamin D levels is an important step forward in preventative care and correct and supervised supplementation could have an important impact on our health. In my quest for reason and balance and as far as the sun is concerned my preference is to sit out in the sun whenever the opportunity occurs usually for about 30 minutes until there is slight pinkness and then cover up to avoid burning.

Things Are Never Simple

How much vitamin D your body actually makes depends on a number of factors.
The angle of the sun
- Where you are in the world (on the Equator or Northern Europe)
- Whether it is winter, summer, spring or autumn
- What time of day it is, with the midday sun obviously offering the strongest rays
Your ethnic grouping
- Those, say of Indian or African descent with darker skins are more susceptible to deficiency in Vitamin D living in northern climates compared to fairer skinned individuals.
- For darker skinned individuals more exposure to the sun is required to gain adequate amounts of the vitamin.
Altitude
- Are you up a mountain where the rays are stronger?
Your Age
- The older you get the less your body is able to make vitamin D from the sun
How Much Skin is Exposed
- Are you in a burqa or a bikini!

Vitamin D Council Recommended Intake For Vitamin D in International Units (IU)
Infants and Children: 1000IU – 2000IU maximum
Adults: 5000IU – 10,000IU maximum
To put these recommendations into context your body can produce 10,000-25,000IU Vitamin D after just a short time of full body sun exposure. Vitamin D is fat-soluble and supplements should be consumed with meals with fat of some sort.

Vitamin K2

Most people and even some doctors have never heard of Vitamin K2. Vitamin K1 the blood clotting vitamin was discovered in 1929 by a German scientist and its letter comes from Koagulationsvitamin. The two K vitamins are very different. K1 is found in plant foods and K2 is found in animal sources and fermented foods.

There is much excitement surrounding Vitamin K2. It has largely gone un-noticed and much more research needs to take place and clinical evidence gathered but the growing belief today is that:

Vitamin K2 plays a crucial role in directing calcium to bones in synergy with Vitamin D. Importantly, it also prevents the build up of calcium in soft tissue (calcification) such as the arteries that can lead to arterial plaque leading to strokes and heart attacks.

In the past the higher prevalence of fermented foods would have meant more intake of Vitamin K2. Today supplementation is being advised by some for its strong association with possible reduction in heart disease.[46]

6. STRESS, BABOONS AND BRITISH CIVIL SERVANTS

We all keep being told that stress is bad but we do not really take the fact on board. On my journey of discovery I have read quite a lot about stress but the message never really sank in until I found a National Geographic/Stanford University documentary on the work of Stanford University, Neurobiologist Robert Sapolsky and also of Sir Michael Marmot Professor of Epidemiology and Public Health at University College London.(47)

These two individuals were carrying out similar studies in totally different parts of the world. Sapolsky was carrying out a study on the effect of social stress on baboons in Africa. Professor Marmot meanwhile was looking at the social stress of British civil servants.

It transpires that baboons, apart from having to focus on eating for 3 hours a day in order to get their required calories, do not have to worry about anything very much. Not having much to do, however, is pretty bad news. The community of baboons that Sapolsky studied spent most of their spare time "bothering" each other. A lot of tortuous, bullying behaviour took place and depending on where the baboons were in the social pecking order resulted in different levels stress being experienced.

Needless to say the alpha males at the top of the pecking order were doing a lot of the bullying but not receiving anything back. They were in control of their situation and experienced no stress. The baboons lower down the pecking order never knew what to expect next …. From being pounced on, to having their hair pulled to worse – they were constantly in a heightened state of awareness and felt little control over their own situation.

What Sapolsky went on to discover, was really quite shocking. He carried out tests on his community of baboons and looked closely at the state of their arteries. The relationship between position in the hierarchy and narrowing of the arteries due to atheroschlerosis was consistent. Those in the top echelons were fit and well and had clear, healthy arteries. As you moved down the social scale the level of "clogging" of the arteries increased and in addition weight also became an issue.

Even more concerning was that when they did comparative studies of the primates' brains, more data came out to support the social strata theory. Brain atrophy (shrinkage) was also apparent leading to reduction in the cognitive behaviour of those primates lower down the social ladder.

Baboons Don't Smoke

The beauty of the study on baboons was that it was able to remove certain factors that might muddy the waters when looking at effects of stress on the human body. Baboons do not drink alcohol, they do not smoke and they all eat, pretty much, the same diet.

Perceived Control Over Your Existence Is Important

Professor Marmot's study that had spanned 40 years, looking at 28,000 British civil servants came to similar conclusions.

The British civil service has a very rigid hierarchical employment ranking system. Again, like in the baboon community the civil servants at the top felt much more in control over their existence than those at the bottom. Being able to observe so many people over such a time period, individuals who would have similar health care benefits and education was very valuable. Marmot observed that ranking "intimately related to risk of disease and length of life".

Whatever your view is on this research the main thing to take away is that stress …. Is really bad and should be managed as much as possible. The perceived and imperceived physiological impact it has on our body cannot be underestimated. Stress will make you want to eat, hungry or not. Eating the wrong foods will only heighten anxiety and make the situation worse, whilst the right foods will minimise negative feelings.

Always remember exercise is a good stress reliever. Finding techniques to manage stress, to suit our needs, is vital.

7. SLEEP IS A POWER TOOL FOR HEALTH

Whatever we do, we must be sure to nurture and protect good quality sleep at night. Eight hours seems to be considered optimal. When we sleep our body:
- Rests
- Protects our hormone function
- Enhances our immunity
- Is rebalancing brain chemicals
- Heals
- Stores our memories
- Is busy repairing blood vessels
- Is eliminating toxins
- Keeps our hunger in check (lack of sleep can increase the Ghrelin hormone)
- Reduces our risk of high blood pressure, diabetes, heart and kidney disease.

Or in other words, if we don't sleep well, none of these vital protective functions can be carried out properly and we severely increase our risk of ill health. We must find the resolve to remove all electronics not only from our bedrooms but especially, if we are to do our duty and protect them, from our childrens' bedrooms. Even if they are protected from the cyber world, sleep disruption will affect everyone who is using these gadgets. Effectively firing up the brain just before closing their eyes to try to go to sleep.

8. THE POWER OF EXERCISE

Regular exercise is absolutely fundamental to maintaining health. In addition and notably aerobic exercise has the power to stimulate the growth of new brain cells a process called neurogenisis. In addition memory is enhanced by regular, short sessions of exercise that raise your heartbeat.

Exercise helps combat chronic inflammation thus helping to ward off disease. As always though, in the pursuit of reason and balance, keep an eye on 'wear and tear'. Pounding the pavements on a regular basis may be good for your heart but what effect will it have on your knee joints in the long-term? Ensure that you vary your exercise and avoid repetitive movements that impact your joints. With antibiotic resistance becoming more prevalent, in the future hip and knee joint operations may not be so run of the mill as they are today…. So look after them!

9. INTERMITTENT FASTING

Intermittent fasting seems to produce some very good results and there are many books on the topic. The main benefits described in clinical reports are:

1. Improves your sensitivity to Insulin and Leptin
2. Its potential for slowing bone mineral density loss
3. Assists repair of DNA
4. Enhances cognitive performance
5. Can increase lifespan
6. Decreases abdominal fat
7. Decreases inflammation
8. Its potential to rejuvenate the immune system
9. Reduces the risk factors that contribute to diabetes, heart disease, cancer and aging.

That said, it must be highlighted that intermittent fasting is not suitable for everyone especially growing children, pregnant women, mothers who are breast-feeding and type 1 diabetics. If embarking on intermittent fasting it is even more important to eat fresh, healthy, nutritious food.

There are many different ways to fast intermittently but two methods in particular are: 1. Eating normally (within moderation) 5 days a week and then have 2 consecutive days when only 600 calories are consumed (for women) and 800 calories are consumed (for men).
        2. Alternatively some people find that they are more comfortable with restricting their daily meals to only two meals a day and having them within a 6-8 hour window; choosing to either have breakfast and lunch or lunch and dinner. This enables them to fast daily for 16-18 hours over a 24 hour period.

There are more challenging versions such as a 5 day fast studied by Dr Valter Longo. His work is continuing at the University of Southern California and he is someone to watch as he goes on to produce more detailed results.(48)

CHAPTER FOUR
SOME OTHER THINGS TO THINK ABOUT

1. REASON AND BALANCE

An approach of reason and balance is essential when it comes to health and nutrition. Remembering always that our body works holistically and not as independent organs and systems.

Fads
We must resist jumping on the latest bandwagon that focuses too much in one direction and is hailed as the ultimate solution to health and weight issues:
Calorie Restriction Diet
High Protein Diet
High Fat Low Carb Diet
Low Fat High Carb Diet
Veganism
Vegetarianism
Paleo
Fruitarian Diet, etc, etc

In my quest for reason and balance I believe we should return to the way of eating prior to the "marketing men" and the industrial farms. Similar to the way our grand parents and great grand parents may well have eaten. Always though, with the emphasis on fresh vegetables in particular.

2. DIVERSITY AND MODERATION

These two words sum up, in a nutshell, what is good for us but many people's diets no longer reflect either of these characteristics.

Even those who are keen to eat healthily may tend to fixate on certain things ... Don't eat kale everyday ... instead focus on a variety of different greens and salads and add variety and interest to such plates with items such as garlic, onions, eggs, seeds, herbs, spices, other vegetables, pre and probiotic foods etc.

Try also to alternate the sources of your food i.e. don't necessarily always buy your broccoli from the same place.

3. MEDICINE A SCIENCE OF SEPARATE PARTS?

We have tended to look at the subject of the body and human health in pockets. Doctors specialise in organs or specific areas of the body. Yet maybe a more holistic approach is needed as the body is so inter-connected.

For example mental conditions are now recognised to be intricately associated with the state of the gut. Does a psychiatrist ever question or suggest to a patient to simultaneously seek advice on their intestinal health as part of the process? Probably not.

In the same way much of the research on vitamins has been conducted in isolation of one another. However, all our essential vitamins and minerals work closely together and need each other in order to carry out their beneficial function.

Misuse of Medications Can Rob Us of Our Nutrients and Our Health

We are encouraged, by some in the medical community and advertising to take a mountain of medication. Older generations may have reminded us to dress warmly, wear a hat, have some broth and an early night if you were at a low ebb. They were the generation who remembered a time before antibiotics and fever-lowering medication, when getting run down or catching a chill could become a little more serious.... We rely on our meds so we do not take care, but we use them liberally at our peril.

By being so ready to resort to medication we can expose ourselves to side effects that can often lead to worse conditions than those initially treated. For example many basic medications can have serious long-term impact on our intestine, damaging the fine balance of beneficial bacteria that we are now discovering plays such an important part in protecting our health in the first place.

In addition our valuable nutrients are taken up to metabolise these drugs adding further to our nutrient deficiencies. Thus our medications can create further problems whilst only patching symptoms and offering no cure.

102

Vets Versus Doctors

If our pet is ill and we take it to the vet you will not be surprised if the vet asks you what your pet has been eating. You will view it as a thoroughly reasonable question for the vet to ask. When was the last time a doctor asked you that question? They probably would not want to be so bold! Still today nutrition is a subject that is barely included in medical training.

The inclination of medicine in recent years has not been about prevention instead it seems to have focused on 'cure' but not necessarily on the cure of the condition. Instead on cure of the symptoms that is an entirely different approach.

Doctors have been inclined and equally pressurized by patients to offer quick solutions and so called 'magic bullets' – pills that can be easily taken to immediately alleviate symptoms and discomfort without looking at cause.

So we have seen a culture of over-prescription that has lead to antibiotic misuse and a sea of pills that so often cause us further problems and sometimes much more suffering and disease.

We are all beginning to observe the reality of the situation, especially in America, where despite taking the greatest amount of medication than anywhere else in the world, adults and children seem to be suffering illness more and more.

The importance of nutrition when not confused with 'diets' seems to be taking hold with many people ....and doctors .... Who often see their own patients improve through the individuals' attempts to reverse their condition with targeted, wholesome food.

"The art of medicine consists in amusing the patient
whilst nature cures the disease" Voltaire

"Nutrition is the Medicine of the Future"
Twice Nobel Prize Winner Linus Pauling

The Risk To Our Health From So Many Medications

The incredibly complex inter relationship of nutrients in foods in our bodies begs the question of how we can be happy to take as much medication as we do? How can we possibly know what knock on effects the prescriptions we take really have on our bodies.

Heartburn and Acid Reflux

This is a controversial example where a condition is treated with medication that only eases the symptoms. The medication in fact goes on to perpetuate the initial condition thus continuing the need for the medication.(49)

In summary the theory works as follows:

-       Our lifestyle is such that we perhaps eat bigger portions than we ought to. So then we feel overly full.
-       We slump on the sofa with a full stomach.
-       The pressure of the food in the stomach causes some of the stomach contents (including some stomach acid) to be pushed up into the oesophagus where the lining is too sensitive to withstand the hydrochloric acid from the stomach.
-       Heartburn ensues.
-       Antacid medications are then taken to neutralise the acid in the stomach to stop it burning when it comes back up into the oesophagus again.
-       BUT THEN …. The acidity in the stomach is reduced. This prevents food from being sufficiently broken down and at the same time allows bad bugs (that prefer a less acid environment) to multiply in the stomach.
-       These bugs go on to feed off the poorly or undigested food thus allowing them to multiply further.
-       The bi-product of their feeding is gas that accumulates in the stomach and produces bloating.
-       The bloating causes pressure in the stomach that leads to more acidity being pushed up into the oesophagus causing more heartburn.

- Leading to the need for more antacids…
- So the anti acids alleviate the discomfort but aggravate the overall condition that can lead to more severe problems down the line.
- Antacids may have their place but like so much they are prescribed and purchased indiscriminately and overall may become more of a problem than a solution.

Bad Science

Can Big Money And Good Science Really Mix?

The Funding of Biased Science?

Back in the 1920s and 30s there was, it could be argued, a golden age of research work and understanding of nutrition. For example the B Vitamins were identified between 1912 and 1937, Vitamin D in 1922, Vitamin C was isolated and synthesised in 1932-34.

That period in time, however, could be seen as the twilight of uninfluenced research in universities. From then on there was more funding and subsequent control of universities by large companies.

Commercial influence will have undoubtedly had an affect on the type of research and the results and conclusions.

More and more science has been built on this work. With many scientific papers being produced there is a tendency to only read the summaries or "abstracts". This leaves all the important quirks and caveats and possible mistakes of the actual experiments and their results buried deep in the heart of the science papers leaving the real science ignored and misunderstood and bad science to escape criticism.

Today Archived Research is Available To All

The loading of archived research that is now available to people all over the world has led to a considerable amount of reviewing of data. For example "Google Scholar" is worth exploring or being aware of and "PubMed" specializes in reviews of clinical research, with summaries and full technical reports. It comprises 24 million biomedical citations. Included is work done in 1890s-1940s by the scientific community when it was still relatively "pharmaceutical /food industry influence-free".

During this period there was interest and understanding that food choices could strongly affect the gut and physical and mental health. However, the pharmaceutical industry's rapid growth, over the 20th century resulted in a move away from this "unsophisticated" approach to health and was predominantly discarded by the established medical community.

A lot of precious, fundamental science attributed to this period has been ignored in recent history.

4. CONFUSED AND MIS-INFORMED?

The confusion starts at the top with important institutions and public Authorities and encompasses the rest of us as the confusion of the drip, drip feed of information and contradiction has left people disinterested and detached for it seems impossible to make any sense of things.

We Won't Be Seeing Adverts For Spinach Or Kale Anytime Soon!

Promoting food through established channels such as mainstream TV and advertising is a very expensive business. Marketing of this nature is usually only afforded by large companies such as food and pharmaceutical companies. In reality we are influenced so much by the one sided, continual messages streaming into our homes at night on TV. These adverts that are part of our everyday life give us a sense of safe, established knowledge. These industries have a vested interest in maintaining things as they are.

Who will tell the other side of the story? Relying on advertising revenue, commercial media may tend to limit how controversial it is in terms of voicing arguments that do not support the food and pharmaceutical industries that will no doubt be some of their main sources of income.

If we are to really address modern day sickness and obesity then there is a huge science based debate to be had with a need for freedom to question established knowledge without being branded as incompetent, foolish or dishonest. I believe that debate is finally starting as more people are becoming informed, courtesy, partly to the internet.

Medicine And Money

Money has also created an imbalance in medicine toward drugs for masking symptoms and pain rather than understanding food to understand cause. The problem is you can't patent food

The UK is Lucky to Have the NHS

Fortunately in the UK the NHS succumbs, to an extent, to different pressures (being cost driven and not profit driven) and may not suffer the apparent imbalance existing in the US where a much greater proportion of medicine is funded through health insurance and implemented through private practice. This has allowed health care to become extremely big business that may not necessarily put the emphasis on patient welfare but on profits instead.

Anyone for Golf?

In the US pharmaceutical companies blatantly woo doctors in order to encourage them to prescribe their drugs to their patients. Heart disease is one of the USA's biggest industries from medication through to surgery and all the stages in between! Even the literature that doctor's read to keep up to date ….on medication mainly, is often written and funded by pharmaceutical companies as are the conferences that doctors attend.

Recommending Ibuprofen or Turmeric?

I am certainly not an advocate for shunning pharmaceuticals completely. They have their place and I certainly benefited from receiving pharmaceutical treatment to stabilise my rheumatoid arthritis initially. It not only managed my pain but it stopped further joint damage occurring. It gave me the time to change my eating habits and get to grips with the inflammatory causes.

However, with doctors more up to speed on the functions of medication rather than the nutrients in food they are more likely to prescribe medication for joint pain than give tips on pro and anti inflammatory foods. But if doctors understood their vitamins and minerals and appreciated food as intricately as they know their drugs we would all be a lot healthier.

"Pay The Farmer Now Or Pay The Doctor Later"

This is an expression that has become more prevalent in America recently – where they have allowed profit to dominate in so much of their farming at the expense of quality and nutritional value of the food that is produced. Realising what is happening some Americans are warning that food choice is boiling down to having to understand that if we insist on wanting food at the cheapest possible price then we will pay later with our health.

In fact the amount of cheap processed food that is consumed as an alternative to more expensive quality whole foods often works out as costing more for the individual. This is due to the sheer addictive nature of the food, the desire for much larger quantities and the medication taken later to patch the negative symptoms created by the food.

The UK is currently witnessing the struggle that dairy farmers are having in order to get paid enough for milk production. The last thing we want is to lose those dairy farms that allow their cows to be partly pasture raised/grass fed.

5. SO WHAT IS THE RIGHT BALANCE – WHAT SHOULD WE EAT?

Carbohydrates? Protein? Fat?

These are the three 'macro nutrients' that humans are able to eat and give us the energy and vitamins, minerals and antioxidants that we need for good health.

We have got ourselves into a fluster over these fundamental food categories in the last few decades.

I do not think there is one answer to what ratio of these foods we should eat and anyway it depends on our age, whom we are and what we do. There are, however, a few issues to flag up that should be taken into account and we will hear them being discussed more and more as time moves forward:

1. **Carbohydrate** is a word that encompasses too many very different types of food and we need to separate them out. What are they:

Sugar, Refined Carbohydrates, Whole grains, Legumes, Vegetables & Fruit.

Sugar, fructose without fibre, grains and whole grains and sugar producing starchy carbohydrates such as potatoes and rice are the foods that will have the biggest impact on raising your blood sugar levels and go towards increasing your insulin resistance.

As your insulin resistance increases your liver will make more and more sugar and fat. This in turn increases the amount of sugar and fat in your blood, increases your blood triglyceride levels causing more body and tummy fat to be stored. It leads to high blood pressure and all the other health issues we have covered earlier.
So ….
- **Sugar** is obviously a no no.
- **Refined carbohydrates**, we are told are bad news too. (Anything with refined flour).

- **Legumes**, some will argue, should be avoided altogether but nothing is ever that black and white. They are rich in fibre so will not raise your blood sugars significantly but legumes contain what are known as the anti-nutrients: lectin and phytic acid or phytates.
  - o Lectin can have the potential to cause health problems but if you tolerate legumes (eg do not trigger bloating or discomfort) then they can probably be consumed in moderation once or twice a week. Lectin can be mostly removed through soaking of beans for example.
  - o Phytic acid. Some get very worked up because of the fact that it binds to certain minerals also contained within the food item and prevents mineral absorption (in particular zinc and iron). Phytic acid can also interfere with our digestive enzymes. However new research suggests that phytic acid may have some benefits as an antioxidant (preventing the formation of free radicals). It may also prevent the accumulation of heavy metals and enhance intercellular communication.(49a)

    In summary, therefore, we can say, here too, the jury is out … but legumes are a very good source of fibre and a very good way to raise your Bacteriodetes (see page 59).

- **Whole grains** - Our shift toward grain consumption has maybe gone too far and this can have an impact on our on going battle to minimise insulin resistance. I believe that this may be largely due to our grain consumption being on top of an already, overly high sugar consumption.

  For me - there is only so much I can eat in a day and I want to make sure that it is as nutrient dense and fibre packed as possible. So I would rather fill up on nutritious and healthy vegetables and a little fruit. I do, however, like porridge oats for breakfast occasionally, especially on busy days. They do not naturally contain gluten (other than possible cross contamination in the milling process). Oats are high in fibre but sugar spikes can also be minimised by consuming porridge with a spoonful of flaxseed, a little butter, or full fat yoghurt or some coconut oil. I like mine with cinnamon too.

Yet foods made from grains such as bread have a comfort element to them and some may feel it is too miserable to exist without it. I loved my bread but I no longer have it and no longer miss it. I certainly no longer miss the immediate bloating and general discomfort I felt after eating bread, pizza or a plate of pasta. Instead I enjoy, and sometimes simply feel the need for, a bit of good old starchy food. Roast potatoes or a delicious bowl of rice (yes white rice!) cooked in chicken stock. Consumed in moderation and combined within a meal of fibrous vegetables and a little protein and fat to help minimise the starchy foods' effect on blood sugars. When allowed to cool to room temperature, both white rice and potatoes gain healthy levels of resistant starch that is a beneficial food for intestinal microbes. The Mediterranean diet often features cold potatoes served with olive oil and herbs.

There is great division on the topic of whole grains but there is a growing number of researchers who believe that when advice changed in the middle of the 20th century to consume less fat, the increased emphasis on grains that came about led to many health problems. This of course includes, in part, the gluten factor and why, with many questions raised about it, but not many answered, I choose to avoid gluten (not completely, though, in case I build up an unnecessarily serious intolerance).[50]

A leading researcher on the subject is Dr Alessio Fasano (see the recommended reading list at the back of the book. There are also a number of lectures uploaded onto You Tube, given by him on the subject of gluten and how it could be affecting many more people than just those diagnosed with Coeliac Disease.)

- **Fibrous vegetables and fruit (such as berries – lower fructose, higher fibre)** are brilliant, offering fibre in all its forms and brimming with vitamins, minerals and antioxidants (phytonutrients). We should eat more of them in all their colours ….It is a question of balance, but the scales are best tipped toward vegetables and some fruit. Nuts and seeds should be consumed in moderation as nature intended.

- **Experiment for yourself.** Excluding foods for a period of time is the best way to assess whether certain types of foods affect you or not.

-

2. Fat - is a complicated tale but in summary, the questioning of established guidelines has lead to the following points being highlighted many times by different authors:

- Taking animal fats out of our diets has certainly made our food less tasty.
- To correct this, sugar was added by food manufacturers, with disastrous effect.
- Inflammatory polyunsaturated fats were promoted to replace saturated fat.
- At the same time refined grain/cereal consumption was encouraged reducing our overall nutrient intake and if you take Dr Perlmutter's message from his book "Grain Brain"; the fats removed had helped to enhance our cognitive function and the grains that were encouraged, reduce our cognitive function.
- The highly rated Mediterranean diet uses predominantly monounsaturated fat from olive oil, also ample amounts of fish and its omega 3 oil is prominent in the diet and the Mediterranean's did not, traditionally, shy away from animal fat, using far more of the animal than we do today. Polyunsaturated fat did not feature in high quantities.

Saturated fat has an important place in our diet and we may well have suffered from avoiding it and/or substituting it with less than ideal alternatives. …. Be wary though of the next wave of emphatic advice ….that high fat diets allow us to be in perpetual fat burning mode, offering us a heightened cognitive state, endurance energy and longevity. It sounds wonderful and may be it is true but it is extreme and the point is we just do not know. With the new emphasis being placed on the microbiome we are discovering that we are all different and our gut bacteria is significantly influenced by our immediate environment. Switching to a high fat diet may not necessarily create an ideal balance of bacteria in our intestine … but these are questions that are only now being addressed more frequently in science (see back to the Burkina Faso study on page 59).

Certainly, those researching the microbes in our gut believe that, for their healthy balance, fibre is the way forward and most of us are just simply not getting enough.

That said eating more high quality fat helps maintain satiety and is a good energy source.

Quality sources:

Olive oil	Coconut oil	Butter and eggs	Grass fed meats and their fats
Avocados	Olives	Raw nuts (in moderation)	

3. Protein The discussion on protein has similar issues. Certain diets in the last few years have placed a lot of positive emphasis on a higher consumption of protein in our diet. Either to lose weight or because this was the 'natural' way to eat like our Paleolithic fore fathers. However if Dr Valter Longo's work in Southern California, is anything to go by then we should be wary of too much animal protein consumption, especially in mid-life due to the possible increased risks it may cause in promoting tumour growth.

Personally I am enjoying food more than ever and what I eat has never been tastier thanks to a renewed focus on herbs and spices and delicious animal fat. Meat and fish remains important but there is, I think, a fine line between too much meat and too little that can lead to malnourishment. So meat and fish are small side servings on my plate of vegetables, topped with a good helping of healthy fats to keep the brain in shape, the body functioning well and to ensure that I can absorb all those lovely fat soluble vitamins.

Wild Recommendations

With everything seemingly in a state of flux I would love to see our amazing health service system in the UK lead the world in changing the nature of front line care. GP surgeries could be given a major role in nutritional advice and education and possibly even look at tailored supplementation for effective preventative care. Vitamin D education, for example, might have a massive impact on the nation's health. (Government policy in the 1940s saw children being given cod liver oil... a rich source of Vitamin D.)

If doctors were more in tune with the possible deficiencies and toxicities that are at the root of most diseases they could emphasize the possible underlying causes and could steer patients toward self-help advice and approved website links for better nutrition.

The internet is full of medical and nutritional sites recommending all sorts of things. Some recommendations are wild and even dangerous, others are sensible. Whatever they are though, they are obviously symptomatic of a need for answers and more help than we are currently getting from our doctors in our quest for well-being.

Many of the scientific advances that are being made are, in all aspects of medicine, simply fantastic. Doctors, specialists and surgeons have skills and techniques available to them that are formidable. I believe we can obtain similar bold achievements at a preventative and educational end of medicine. After all where does the word doctor come from – the Latin verb *docēre* meaning "to teach".

Food, Emotion, Discipline, Routine and Projects!!

- Food is very much linked to emotion. There are those who like to reward themselves with food when they have achieved something. There are those who resort to food when things do not go well. Yet the link between food and emotion is much tighter when one is still addicted to sugar. Break that link first of all and at least our hormones will not be working against us and we have a chance of moving forward and achieving more.
- Procrastination equals misery! Misery may lead to eating naughty things... A little bit of discipline will help us tackle the jobs we dislike first. Then we are free to get on with the rest of our day or week with a lighter load on our shoulders.
- Reflect on changes that could be made to improve the daily routine; incorporate them slowly.
- Take time to sit down with a notebook and keep a running list of the things that need to be done but also a list of things to arrange to look forward to.
- Regularly take a moment to look up a few more simple and tasty recipes to prepare.
- Place more value on your time and reassess how you spend your time.
- Have a project on the go that you look forward to returning to.
- .... and make sure you always have a reason to jump out of bed in the morning even when you're 90.

Conviviality

Let us not forget this wonderful part of life as we sink deeper into the virtual world! In striving to make food "convenient" we may have lost sight of its potential to be at the centre of a world that brings together friends, family, communication, laughter, music and conviviality.

We should embrace the need to cook and eat wholesome good food that we prepare with love and attention. Thought and consideration in the planning can make the preparation of a meal far easier than we might think. Gatherings can be more frequent if they are easy and if everyone prepares and brings a dish. It will produce meals with more variety.

A far cry from a pre-prepared meal on the sofa, in front of the TV ....

Chaos Of The Universe

I have often thought about the chaos in the Universe and how much of what happens is random. The fact that we have managed to create as much order as we have on our little planet is a marvel. What I'm trying to say is there is, as always, a balance between empowerment, belief that we can change and improve our health through nutrition and a pursuit of ultimate control that can take over your life and not necessarily lead to a happy existence.

I saw a couple on TV who had been pursuing a severe calorie restriction diet for years in order to achieve longevity but the pursuit of this goal had created the bleakest of lifestyles and they turned out to be the oldest looking 60 year olds I had ever seen!

So we must try our best to eat well but be careful not to obsess and get bogged down with trying to find the ultimate way of eating because there is no 'one way'.

There are so many people out there so radically convinced of the ultimate solutions but they do not necessarily work for you.

Whoever you are though, I believe:

- When we look at the money we have to spend, if we can, we should prioritise the best quality food we can afford for ourselves and our family.

- In the end it will be our united and informed purchasing power that will change things for the better and we must be prepared to spend if we are to maintain the quality of our food. If we opt for the cheap choices now we will pay with our health later.

  … and finally:

- Sugar destroys health

- Chronic inflammation is our enemy and

- Whole foods have magnificent power to rebuild health

Eat a good variety of fresh food
Don't be afraid of precious healthy fats
Keep moving
Nurture good sleeping habits
Moderation in all things
Manage stress and
Be happy and compassionate

Happier
Healthier
Achievers
Into Old Age

Further Recommended Reading

- Dr Martin Blaser: author of "Missing Microbes"
- Sarah Boseley: Guardian newspapers award winning Health Editor and author of "The Shape We're In: How Junk Food and Diets Are Shortening Our Lives"
- Dr Natasha Campbell McBride: Masters in Neurology and Nutrition and author of "Gut and Psychology Syndrome" and "Put Your Heart in Your Mouth"
- Dr Carolyn Dean – researcher and author "The Magnesium Miracle"
- Sally Fallon: President of the Weston A Price Foundation and author of "Nourishing Traditions"
- Dr Alessio Fasano:Italian medical doctor, pediatric gastroenterologist and researcher. Chair of Pediatrics at Harvard Medical School
- Ben Goldacre author of "Bad Science" and "Bad Pharma"
- Dr Stephan Guyenet: obesity researcher, neurobiologist, and author. Bachelor of Science in biochemistry (University of Virginia) and a PhD in neurobiology (University of Washington). "Whole Health Source- Nutrition and Health Science" blog.
- Wardeh Harmon – author of "The Complete Idiot's Guide to Fermenting Foods"
- Patrick Holford – author of "The Optimum Nutrition Bible"
- Dr Richard Johnson – author of "The Fat Switch"
- Dr Malcolm Kendrick – author of "The Cholesterol Con" and "Doctoring Data: How to sort out medical advice from medical nonsense"
- Chris Kresser – Health researcher, author and blogger "chriskresser.com" has 250,000 followers
- Dr Robert Lustig – author of "Fat Chance"
- Chris Masterjohn PhD in Nutritional Sciences at City University of New York. Author of blog called "The Daily Lipid"
- Linus Pauling Twice Nobel Prize Winner. Author of "Vitamin C and the Common Cold"
- Dr David Perlmutter: Board Certified Neurologist and Fellow of the American College of Nutrition. Author of New York Times No. 1 best seller

"Grain Brain" and "Brain Maker"
- Weston A Price Foundation website
- Monica Reinagel – Masters in Human Nutrition, Board Certified nutrition specialist. Author of "The Inflammation Free Diet Plan"
- Jo Robinson – author of "Eating on the Wild Side: A radical new way to select and prepare foods to reclaim the nutrients and flavour we've lost"
- Gene Stone: New York Times No. 1 best seller author of "Forks Over Knives" and "The Secrets of People Who Never Get Sick"
- Gary Taubes: American author of Nobel Dreams, Bad Science: The Short Life and Weird Times of Cold Fusion, and Good Calories, Bad Calories, titled The Diet Delusion in the UK and Australia

References

1. WITH ANY LUCK WE ARE ON THE BRINK OF A FOOD REVOLUTION
Reversing Type 2 Diabetes through diet.
Dr. Sarah Hallberg is the medical director and founder of the Indiana University-Arnett Health Medical Weight Loss Program. She created the program around 2012 and since then it has helped hundreds of patients reverse and prevent type 2 diabetes through low carb and high fat nutrition.
http://www.diabetes.co.uk/blog/2015/05/ignore-the-guidelines-eat-low-carb-and-high-fat-dr-sarah-hallberg-on-how-to-reverse-type-two-diabetes/

Type 2 Diabetes Etiology and reversibility Roy Taylor, MD, FRCP
Author Affiliations Magnetic Resonance Centre, Institute of Cellular Medicine, Newcastle University, Newcastle upon Tyne, U.K. Corresponding author: Roy Taylor, roy.taylor@ncl.ac.uk.
http://care.diabetesjournals.org/content/36/4/1047.full

2. WITHIN A WHISPER OF TRIGGERING ILLNESS
Food as Exposure: Nutritional Epigenetics and the New Metabolism
http://www.palgrave-journals.com/biosoc/journal/v6/n2/full/biosoc20111a.html
Dr D Perlmutter – Brain Maker Published by Little, Brown and Company April 2015

3. SUGAR UNWRAPPED – INCREASE IN SUGAR CONSUMPTION
http://wholehealthsource.blogspot.co.uk/2012/02/by-2606-us-diet-will-be-100-percent.html
Stephan Guyenet Obesity researcher, neurobiologist, and author. BS in biochemistry (University of Virginia) and a PhD in neurobiology (University of Washington).

4. METABOLIC SYNDROME
www.ncbi.nlm.nih.gov/pubmed/17921363
by RJ Johnson - 2007 - Cited by 491 - Related articles
Potential role of sugar (fructose) in the epidemic of hypertension, obesity and the metabolic syndrome, diabetes, kidney disease, and cardiovascular disease. ... may be a major mechanism by which fructose can cause cardiorenal disease.

5. SUGAR, FRUCTOSE, FRUIT – SORTING OUT THE CONFUSION

http://www.nature.com/nrgastro/journal/v7/n5/full/nrgastro.2010.41.html

"The role of fructose in the pathogenesis of NAFLD and the metabolic syndrome" Jung Sub Lim, Michele Mietus-Snyder, Annie Valente, Jean-Marc Schwarz & Robert H. Lustig

Dr R Lustig "Fat Chance" Published by Fourth Estate in October 2014

http://ajprenal.physiology.org/content/290/3/F625.short

"A causal role for uric acid in fructose-induced metabolic syndrome" Takahiko Nakagawa, Hanbo Hu, Sergey Zharikov, Katherine R. Tuttle, Robert A. Short, Olena Glushakova, Xiaosen Ouyang, Daniel I. Feig, Edward R. Block, Jaime Herrera-Acosta, Jawaharlal M. Patel, Richard J. Johnson
American Journal of Physiology - Renal Physiology Published 1 March 2006 Vol. 290 no. 3, F625-F631 DOI: 10.1152/ajprenal.00140.2005

6. FAT STORAGE SYSTEM

Hibernating bear / Fat Storage System
http://www.ncbi.nlm.nih.gov/pmc/articles/PMC3660463/Dr R Johnson

7.FRUCTOSE DOES NOT SUPPRESS GHRELIN

www.ncbi.nlm.nih.gov/pubmed/15181085
by KL Teff - 2004 - Cited by 496 - Related articles
Because fructose, unlike glucose, does not stimulate insulin secretion, we ... but postprandial suppression of ghrelin was significantly less pronounced after HFr ...

8. FRUCTOSE SUPPRESSES THE I'M FULL SIGNAL PEPTIDE YY

"Dietary Sugars and Health" Edited by Michael I Goran, Luc Tappy, Kim-Anne Le. CRC Press Taylor and Francis Group page 198

9. FRUCTOSE SUPPRESSES LEPTIN

www.ncbi.nlm.nih.gov/pubmed/15181085
by KL Teff - 2004 - Cited by 496 - Related articles
Dietary fructose reduces circulating insulin and leptin, attenuates postprandial suppression of ghrelin, and increases triglycerides in women.
TeffKL(1), Elliott SS ...

122

ADDITIONAL REFERENCES FOR SUGAR AND DISEASE
UCSF Mini Medical School for the Public UCTV

Childhood Obesity: Adrift in the "Limbic Triangle"
Michelle L. Mietus-Snyder and Robert H. Lustig
Annual Review of Medicine 59:147-162 (February 2008)

Childhood Obesity: Behavioral Aberration or Biochemical Drive?
Reinterpreting the First Law of Thermodynamics
Robert H. Lustig
Nature Clinical Practice Endocrinology & Metabolism 2(8):447-458 (2006)

Adolescent Overweight and Future Adult Coronary Heart Disease
Kirsten Bibbins-Domingo, Pamela Coxson, Mark T. Pletcher, James Lightwood and Lee Goldman
New England Journal of Medicine, 357(23):2371-2379 (Dec. 6, 2007)

Overweight Adolescents Projected to Have More Heart Disease in Young Adulthood
UCSF News Release, Dec. 5, 2007

Prevalence of Overweight and Obesity in the United States, 1999-2004
Cynthia L. Ogden, Margaret D. Carroll, Lester R. Curtin, Margaret A. McDowell, Carolyn J. Tabak and Katherine M. Flegal
JAMA, 295(13):1549-1555 (April 5, 2006)

chriskresser.com/thyroid-blood-sugar-metabolic-syndrome/
Cached 23 Jul 2010 - **Metabolic syndrome is caused by chronic hyperglycemia (high blood sugar).**

10. FRUCTOSE ON THE LIVER
Journal of Hepatology
Volume 48, Issue 6, June 2008, Pages 993-999
Fructose consumption as a risk factor for non-alcoholic fatty liver disease *
Xiaosen Ouyang[1, †], Pietro Cirillo[1], Yuri Sautin[1], Shannon McCall[2], James L. Bruchette[2], Anna Mae Diehl[3], Richard J. Johnson[1], Manal F. Abdelmalek[3, ,]

123

11. ADDICTION TO FRUCTOSE
www.ingentaconnect.com/content/ben/cdar/2011/00000004/00000003/art00003
The Addiction Potential of Hyperpalatable Foods
Authors: N. Gearhardt, Ashley; Davis, Caroline; Kuschner, Rachel; D. Brownell, Kelly

http://www.sciencedirect.com/science/article/pii/S0149763407000589
Science Direct Elsevier Neuroscience &Biobehavioral Reviews
Volume 32, Issue 1, 2008, Pages 20–39
Authors Nicole M. Avena, Pedro Rada, Bartley G. Hoebel
Evidence for sugar addiction: Behavioral and neurochemical effects of intermittent, excessive sugar intake
[Avena, N.M., Rada, P., Hoebel B.G., 2007.

11a.. IT'S NOT THE FAT – IT'S THE SUGAR
2010 American Society for Nutrition
Meta-analysis of prospective cohort studies evaluating the association of saturated fat with cardiovascular disease[1,2,3,4,5]
   Patty W Siri-Tarino, Qi Sun, Frank B Hu, and Ronald M Krauss
Author Affiliations
   [1]From the Children's Hospital Oakland Research Institute Oakland CA (PWS TRMK) the Departments of Nutrition (QSFBH)Epidemiology (FBH) Harvard School of Public Health Boston MA.

12. WHY SWEETENERS ARE NOT A GOOD IDEA
http://blogs.scientificamerican.com/mind-guest-blog/tricking-taste-buds-but-not-the-brain-artificial-sweeteners-change-braine28099s-pleasure-response-to-sweet/
Tricking Taste Buds but Not the Brain: Artificial Sweeteners Change Brain's Pleasure Response to Sweet

12a. INSULIN RESISTANCE AND BRAIN SHRINKAGE
http://care.diabetesjournals.org/content/36/2/443.short
Insulin Resistance, Brain Atrophy, and Cognitive Performance in Late Middle–Aged Adults

Auriel A. Willette, PHD, GuofanXu, MD, PHD, Sterling C. Johnson, PHD, Alex C. Birdsill, BS, Erin M. Jonaitis, PHD, Mark A. Sager, MD, Bruce P. Hermann, PHD Asenath La Rue, PHD, Sanjay Asthana, MD and Barbara B. Bendlin, PHD

Consequences of Aberrant Insulin Regulation in the Brain: Can Treating Diabetes be Effective for Alzheimer's Disease
http://www.ncbi.nlm.nih.gov/pmc/articles/PMC3263463/

13. INFLAMMATION CAUSE OF MANY MODERN DISEASES
www.cdc.gov/pcd/issues/2012/11_0301.htm
by G Egger - 2012 - Cited by 15 - Related articles
This focus on a predominant cause of infections (ie, microbial pathogens) ultimately led to ... The discovery of a form of low-grade systemic and chronic inflammation ... for many developed countries; approximately 70% of diseases now result from ... These include not only behaviors linked to modern lifestyles facilitated by ...

14. OMEGA 6 AND INFLAMMATION
www.ncbi.nlm.nih.gov/pubmed/12442909
The importance of the ratio of omega-6/omega-3 essential fatty acids.
by AP Simopoulos - 2002 - Cited by 1709 - Related articles
1The Center for Genetics, Nutrition and Health, Washington, DC 20009, USA. cgnh@bellatlantic.net
Excessive amounts of omega-6 polyunsaturated fatty acids (PUFA) and a very ... cardiovascular disease, cancer, and inflammatory and autoimmune diseases, ...
umm.edu/health/medical/altmed/supplement/omega6-fatty-acids
20 Jun 2013.

14a DANGERS OF TRANS FATS
• "Mar 8 2014 FDA filing by HARVARD SCHOOL OF PUBLIC HEALTH – on the Tentative Determination Regarding Partially Hydrogenated Oils; Request for Comments and for Scientific Data and Information"..

14b. EXCESS POLYUNSATURATED FATS CAN LEAD TO CHRONICINFLAMMATION AND DISEASE
Effect of Dietary Fat on Human Breast Cancer Growth and Lung Metastasis in Nude Mice, David P. Rose[*], Jeanne M. Connolly and Carol L. Meschter

15. DEMONIZATION OF BUTTER
Point 1. en.wikipedia.org/wiki/Crisco
Crisco is a brand of shortening produced by The J.M. Smucker Company popular in the United States. Introduced in June 1911 by Procter & Gamble,
Point 6 The Questionable Link Between Saturated Fat and Heart ...
www.wsj.com/.../SB10001424052702303678404579533760760481486 6 May 2014 - Our distrust of saturated fat can be traced back to the 1950s, to a man named Ancel Benjamin Keys, a scientist at the University of Minnesota.
Point 7 "Bad Science" and "Bad Pharma" Books by Ben Goldacre
November 21st, 2009 The Guardian by Ben Goldacre in bad science, big pharma, ... known as The Seven Countries study, where Ancel Keys disregarded all of the countries ...
Point 8 Dietary Fat and Its Relation to Heart Attacks and Strokes
circ.ahajournals.org/content/23/1/133.full.pdf
by IH Page - 1961 - Cited by 102 - Related articles

PROGRAM OF THE AMERICAN HEART ASSOCIATION* ... can Heart Association and is chaired by A. Carnton...Circulation, Volume XXIII, January1961.

15a WHY WE NEED SATURATED FAT
Mary Enig – Westonaprice.org "Benefits of Saturated Fats" Mary Enig attended University of Maryland, College Park (UMCP) MS and PhD in Nutritional Sciences in 1984.From 1984 through 1991, faculty research associate at UMCP with the Lipids Research Group in the Department of Chemistry and Biochemistry, participated in biochemical research on lipids. Licensed Nutritionist in Maryland from May 1988 to October 2008. Master of the American College of Nutrition and former editor of the *Journal of the American College of Nutrition* where she published articles on food fats and oils.[

Board member and the vice president and of the Weston A. Price Foundation
(WAPF) which she co-founded with Sally Fallon in 1999 to promote nutrition and
health advice based on the work of early 20th century dentist and researcher
Weston A. Price.[

16. SATURATED FAT RAISES HDL
J Clin Invest. 1993 Apr; 91(4): 1665–1671. doi: 10.1172/JCI116375
**Dietary fat increases high density lipoprotein (HDL) levels both by increasing
the transport rates and decreasing the fractional catabolic rates of HDL
cholesterol ester** and apolipoprotein (Apo) A-I. Presentation of a new animal
model and mechanistic studies in human Apo A-I transgenic and control mice.
T Hayek, Y Ito, N Azrolan, R B Verdery, K Aalto-Setälä, A Walsh, and J L Breslow
Author information ► Copyright and License information ►

17. SATURATED FATS – ANXIETY, MOOD SWINGS AND VIOLENCE
http://annals.org/article.aspx?articleid=711248
Cholesterol and Violence: Is There a Connection?
Conclusions: A significant association between low or lowered cholesterol levels
and violence is found across many types of studies. Data on this association
conform to Hill's criteria for a causal association. Concerns about increased risk for
violent outcomes should figure in risk–benefit analyses for cholesterol screening
and treatment.

**Assessing the Observed Relationship between Low Cholesterol and
Violence-related Mortality
Implications for Suicide Risk**
• Jay R. Kaplan, Stephen B. Manuck And J. John Mann
Article first published online: 17 DEC 2006
DOI: 10.1111/j.1749-6632.1997.tb52355.x
Issue **Annals of the New York Academy of Sciences**
Volume 836, Neurobiology of Suicide, The: From the Bench to the Clinic pages
57–80, December 1997

18. SATURATED FAT ON BRAIN FUNCTION
Dr D Perlmutter – Brain Maker Published by Little, Brown and Company April 2015

Saturated Fat and Health: Recent Advances in Research
Richard D. Feinman⊠
Lipids. 2010 Oct; 45(10): 891–892.
Published online 2010 Sep 9. doi: 10.1007/s11745-010-3446-8

PMCID: PMC2974200

19. SIZE MATTERS
http://jama.jamanetwork.com/article.aspx?articleid=187669
**Fasting Insulin and Apolipoprotein B Levels and Low-Density Lipoprotein
Particle Size as Risk Factors for Ischemic Heart Disease**

**LDL Particle Number and Risk of Future Cardiovascular Disease in the
Framingham Offspring Study – Implications for LDL Management**
William C. Cromwell, MD,1,2 James D. Otvos, PhD,3 Michelle J. Keyes,
PhD,4,5 Michael J. Pencina, PhD,5 Lisa Sullivan, PhD,6 Ramachandran S. Vasan,
MD,4,7 Peter W.F. Wilson, MD,8 and Ralph B. D'Agostino, PhD4,5
J ClinLipidol. Author manuscript; available in PMC 2009 Aug 4.
Published in final edited form as: J ClinLipidol. 2007 Dec 1; 1(6): 583–592.
doi: 10.1016/j.jacl.2007.10.001

20. IS CHOLESTEROL IN FACT A VITAL ANTIOXIDANT THAT WE NEED MORE
OF AS WE GET OLDER?
http://onlinelibrary.wiley.com/store/10.1111/j.1365-
2753.2011.01767.x/asset/j.1365-
2753.2011.01767.x.pdf?v=1&t=ienyoq1d&s=4253fb04bc497e05b5b059015d1898c
4de2809b0

http://www.ncbi.nlm.nih.gov/pubmed/1937129Another cholesterol hypothesis:
cholesterol as antioxidant

"Putting Your Heart in Your Mouth" – Natural Treatment for Angina,
Atheroschlerosis, Heart Attack, High Blood Pressure, Stroke, Arrhythmia,
Peripheral Vascular Disease – pages 10,15, 18,23,24,27, 30,61.
Author: Dr Natasha Campbell McBride MD MMedSci (neurology), MMedSci
(nutrition).

20a. CHOLESTEROL
http://jama.jamanetwork.com/article.aspx?articleid=1104631
Number of Coronary Heart Disease Risk Factors and Mortality in Patients With First Myocardial Infarction FREE John G. Canto, MD, MSPH; Catarina I. Kiefe, MD, PhD; William J. Rogers, MD; Eric D. Peterson, MD, MPH; Paul D. Frederick, MPH, MBA; William J. French, MD; C. Michael Gibson, MD; Charles V. Pollack, MD, MA; Joseph P. Ornato, MD; Robert J. Zalenski, MD; Jan Penney, RN, MSN; Alan J. Tiefenbrunn, MD; Philip Greenland, MD; for the NRMI Investigators*JAMA*. 2011;306(19):2120-2127. doi:10.1001/jama.2011.1654.

20b. ALTERNATIVE TESTS FOR HEALTH
http://www.ncbi.nlm.nih.gov/pubmed/21388339
Homocysteine: a biomarker in neurodegenerative diseases.
Herrmann W1, Obeid R.
Diseases of the central nervous system are found in patients with severe hyperhomocysteinemia (HHcy). Epidemiological studies show a positive, dose-dependent relationship between mild-to-moderate increases in plasma total homocysteine concentrations (Hcy) and the risk of neurodegenerative diseases, such as Alzheimer's disease, vascular dementia, cognitive impairment or stroke. HHcy is a surrogate marker for B vitamin deficiency (folate, B12, B6) and a neurotoxic agent.

20c. CHOLESTEROL AND LONGEVITY
Uffe Ravnskov, Danish MD and independent researcher.
Journal of the American Geriatrics Society Vol. 59, Issue 10, pages 1779-1785 October 2011.
"Association Between Serum Cholesterol and Non-Cardiovascular Mortality in Older Age".

21.WHAT WILL HAPPEN IN THE FINAL SCENE
"The Great Cholesterol Con" – Author: Dr Malcolm Kendrick (7 July 2008)

"Doctoring the Data" – Author: Dr Malcolm Kendrick

"Putting Your Heart in Your Mouth" – Natural Treatment for Angina, Atueroschlerosis, Heart Attack, High Blood Pressure, Stroke, Arrhythmia, Peripheral Vascular Disease – pages 10,15, 18,23,24,27, 30,61.
Author: Dr Natasha Campbell McBride MD MMedSci (neurology), MMedSci (nutrition).

22. WHICH FATS/OILS TO USE
USDA National Nutrient Database for Standard Reference.The National Agricultural Library
http://ndb.nal.usda.gov/ndb/foods/show/611

23. DEODORISING
Deodorization - AOCS Lipid Library
lipidlibrary.aocs.org/**Oils**Fats/content.cfm?ItemNumber=40326, 27 Jan 2014

24. OUR FEAR OF BUGS COULD BE KILLING US
and
25. AUTOIMMUNE DISEASE AND THE MICROBIOME

"Missing Microbes" Author: Dr Martin Blaser

http://www.actionbioscience.org/genomics/the_human_microbiome.html

Dr D Perlmutter – Brain Maker Published by Little, Brown and Company April 2015

"Gut and Psychology Syndrome" Author: Dr Natasha Campbell McBride MD
MMedSci (neurology), MMedSci (nutrition).
The Economist magazine of August 18, 2012 The human microbiome
Me, myself, us

http://www.sciencedirect.com/science/article/pii/S0165247804000379
Commensal bacteria (normal microflora), mucosal immunity and chronicinflammatory and autoimmune diseases

http://genome.cshlp.org/content/19/12/2317
The NIH Human Microbiome Project

26. GUT/BRAIN AXIS
"Gut and Psychology Syndrome" Author: Dr Natasha Campbell McBride MD MMedSci (neurology), MMedSci (nutrition).

Li, W.; Dowd, S. E.; Scurlock, B.; Acosta-Martinez, V.; Lyte, M. (2009). **"Memory and learning behavior in mice is temporally associated with diet-induced alterations in gut bacteria".** *Physiology & Behavior***96** (4–5): 557–567. doi:10.1016/j.physbeh.2008.12.004. PMID 19135464.

"Gastrointestinal Microflora Studies in Late-Onset Autism".*Clinical Infectious Diseases***35** (Suppl 1): S6–S16. doi:10.1086/341914. PMID 12173102. Finegold, S. M.; Molitoris, D.; Song, Y.; Liu, C.; Vaisanen, M. L.; Bolte, E.; McTeague, M.; Sandler, R.; Wexler, H.; Marlowe, E. M.; Collins, M. D.; Lawson, P. A.; Summanen, P.; Baysallar, M.; Tomzynski, T. J.; Read, E.; Johnson, E.; Rolfe, R.; Nasir, P.; Shah, H.; Haake, D. A.; Manning, P.; Kaul, A. (2002).

"Reduced anxiety-like behavior and central neurochemical change in germ-free mice".*Neurogastroenterology& Motility***23** (3): 255–264, e119.doi:10.1111/j.1365-2982.2010.01620.x. PMID 21054680. Neufeld, K. M.; Kang, N.; Bienenstock, J.; Foster, J. A. (2011).

27. PRESCRIPTIONS FOR ASTHMA
http://www.asthma.org.uk/history

28. CAESARIAN SECTIONS
"Missing Microbes" Author: Dr Martin Blaser Chapter 9 "Mother and Child"

29. THE MOST SIGNIFICANT CONTRIBUTION TO GUT HEALTH IS BELIEVED TO BE FIBRE FROM WHOLE PLANT FOODS AND POLYPHENOLS
http://pubs.acs.org/doi/abs/10.1021/jf2053959
Up-regulating the Human Intestinal Microbiome Using Whole Plant Foods, Polyphenols, and/or Fiber

http://www.phenol-explorer.eu

http://www.ncbi.nlm.nih.gov/pubmed/24452238
Am J ClinNutr. 2014 Mar;99(3):479-89. doi: 10.3945/ajcn.113.074237. Epub 2014 Jan 22.
Flavonoid-rich fruit and vegetables improve microvascular reactivity and inflammatory status in men at risk of cardiovascular disease--FLAVURS: a randomized controlled trial.
Macready AL1, George TW, Chong MF, Alimbetov DS, Jin Y, Vidal A, Spencer JP, Kennedy OB, Tuohy KM, Minihane AM, Gordon MH, Lovegrove JA; FLAVURS Study Group.

30. C DIFFICILE AND FECAL TRANSPLANTS
"Missing Microbes" Author: Dr Martin Blaser

31 FIRMICUTES AND BACTERIODETES
http://www.pnas.org/content/107/33/14691.long
Impact of diet in shaping gut microbiota revealed by a comparative study in children from Europe and rural Africa

32. ALTERING YOUR RATIO
http://www.researchgate.net/profile/George_Fahey/publication/269876705_
Fiber_supplementation_influences_phylogenetic_structure_and_functional_
capacity_of_the_human_intestinal_microbiome_follow-
up_of_a_randomized_controlled_trial/links/54aab4410cf25c4c472f484a.pdf

33. THE MICROBIOME AND OUR GENES
23,000 genes – 3million genes
The Economist magazine of August 18, 2012 The human microbiome

http://www.ncbi.nlm.nih.gov/pmc/articles/PMC3764083/
The Environment Within: Exploring the Role of the Gut Microbiome in Health and Disease, Environ Health Perspect. 2013 Sep; 121(9): A276–A281.

(34) CAUTION AND BALANCE AND A NEW TYPE OF MEDICINE
Chapter 9 – A Forgotten World from "Missing Microbes – How Killing Bacteria Creates Modern Plagues" by Martin Blaser. Published by One World

(35) & (36) FEEDING FOODS REPAIRING FOODS

(35) Protein Promotes Cell Duplication/ Protein Intake and Lifespan

http://www.cell.com/cell-metabolism/abstract/S1550-4131(14)00062-X?_returnURL=http%3A%2F%2Flinkinghub.elsevier.com%2Fretrieve%2Fpii%2FS155041311400062X%3Fshowall%3Dtrue

Low Protein Intake Is Associated with a Major Reduction in IGF-1, Cancer, and Overall Mortality in the 65 and Younger but Not Older Population

(36) Plant Base Food and Cell Repair

Polyphenols: food sources and bioavailability

Claudine Manach, Augustin Scalbert, Christine Morand, Christian Rémésy, and Liliana Jime´

http://ajcn.nutrition.org/content/79/5/727.full#sec-18

Am J ClinNutr May 2004   vol. 79 no. 5 727-747

(37) SPOTLIGHT ON POLYPHENOL PHYTONUTRIENTS AND THE BENEFITS OF PLANT FOODS

2004 American Society for Clinical Nutrition

Polyphenols: food sources and bioavailability

Claudine Manach, AugustinScalbert, Christine Morand, Christian Rémésy, and Liliana Jiménez

(38) TOP TIP TO MAKE YOU TIP TOP

http://www.ncbi.nlm.nih.gov/pubmed/11087546

J Agric Food Chem. 2000 Nov;48(11):5731-5.

Differential inhibition of human platelet aggregation by selected Allium thiosulfinates. Briggs WH1, Xiao H, Parkin KL, Shen C, Goldman IL.

(39) HERBS AND SPICES

Whfoods - Carlsen MH, Halvorsen BL, Holte K et al. The total antioxidant content of more than 3100 foods, beverages, spices, herbs and supplements used worldwide. Nutrition Journal 2010, 9:3 (22 January 2010). 2010

(40) NUTS

http://www.maastrichtuniversity.nl/web/Main/Sitewide/News1/DailyConsumptionOfNutsAndPeanutsLinkedToLowerMortalityRates1.htm

133

(41) WAR
Probiotics and their fermented food products are beneficial for health
1 Helix Pharms Co. Ltd, Kyung-Hee University, and Department of Biological
Sciences of Oriental Medicine, Graduate School of Interdepartmental Studies,
Institute of Oriental Medicines, Kyung-Hee University, Dongdaemoon-gu, Seoul,
Korea
2 PAEC, Islamabad, Pakistan
3 Department of Molecular Biotechnology, Bio/Molecular Informatics Center,
Konkuk University, Gwangjin-gu, Seoul, Korea

http://onlinelibrary.wiley.com/store/10.1111/j.1365-
2672.2006.02963.x/asset/j.1365-
2672.2006.02963.x.pdf;jsessionid=43A71A8277EB5DAAADE3A66CD6392
EFF.f04t01?v=1&t=ifdmy193&s=89d5094582fb63b6601ebd049f8fcb074aa3
be32

42. JUICING OR BLENDING
MolNutr Food Res. 2010 Nov;54(11):1646-58. doi: 10.1002/mnfr.200900580.
**Nonextractable polyphenols, usually ignored, are the major part of dietary
polyphenols: a study on the Spanish diet.**
Arranz S1, Silván JM, Saura-Calixto F.
PMID: 20540148 [PubMed - indexed for MEDLINE]

http://nutritionfacts.org/video/juicing-removes-more-than-just-fiber/
**Polyphenols as dietary fiber associated compounds. Comparative study on
in vivo and in vitro properties**
AccessDenialMessagePlaceholderLaura Bravo, RocioAbia, FulgencioSaura-
Calixto*J. Agric. Food Chem.*, 1994, *42* (7), pp 1481–1487 DOI: 10.1021
/jf00043a017 Publication Date: July 1994

(43) THE MAGNESIUM – CALCIUM RELATIONSHIP IS IMPORTANT
http://www.nutritionalmagnesium.org/calcium-magnesium-balance/

Carolyn Dean MD "The Magnesium Miracle"

(44) IRWIN STONE (1907–1984) was an American biochemist, chemical engineer, and author of "The Healing Factor"
Vitamin C
http://www.vitamincfoundation.org/mega_1_1.html Patrick Holford

(45) VITAMIN D
http://onlinelibrary.wiley.com/doi/10.1111/php.12382/full
Vitamin D and Skin Cancer - Burns - 2014 - Photochemistry and Photobiology - Wiley Online Library

(46) VITAMIN K2
http://jn.nutrition.org/content/134/11/3100.long
Dietary Intake of Menaquinone Is Associated with a Reduced Risk of Coronary Heart Disease: The Rotterdam Study Johanna M. Geleijnse[*,†],Cees Vermeer[**],Diederick E. Grobbee[‡],Leon J. Schurgers[**],Marjo H. J. Knapen[**],Irene M. van der Meer[*], Albert Hofman[*], and Jacqueline C. M. Witteman[*,2]

Dr. Kate Rhéaume-Bleue author of "The Calcium Paradox"

(47) STRESS
https://www.youtube.com/watch?v=eYG0ZuTv5rs
Stress, Portrait of a Killer - Full Documentary (2008) - YouTube

https://www.ucl.ac.uk/whitehallll
University College London – The Stress and Health Study – Whitehall II

(48) INTERMITTENT FASTING
A Periodic Diet that Mimics Fasting Promotes Multi-System Regeneration, Enhanced Cognitive Performance, and Healthspan

http://www.cell.com/cell-metabolism/abstract/S1550-4131(15)00224-7?_returnURL=http%3A%2F%2Flinkinghub.elsevier.com%2Fretrieve%2Fpii%2FS1550413115002247%3Fshowall%3Dtrue

(49) HEARTBURN AND REFLUX AND ANTACIDS
http://link.springer.com/article/10.1016/S1091-255X(00)80032-3
Suppression of gastric acid secretion in patients with gastroesophageal reflux disease results in gastric bacterial overgrowth and deconjugation of bile acids

(49a) POTENTIAL HEALTH BENEFITS OF PHYTIC ACIDS
Potential health benefits and problems associated with antinutrients in foods
Author links open the overlay panel. Numbers correspond to the affiliation list which can be exposed by using the show more link.

- Lilian U. Thompson
  Department of Nutritional Sciences, University of Toronto, Toronto, Ontario, Canada, M5S 1A8, Available online 22 September 2003

(50) SO WHAT IS THE RIGHT BALANCE
GLUTEN - Dr AlessioFasano
http://archinte.jamanetwork.com/article.aspx?articleid=215079&resultclick=1

ABSTRACT
Conclusions Our results suggest that CD occurs frequently not only in patients with gastrointestinal symptoms, but also in first- and second-degree relatives and patients with numerous common disorders even in the absence of gastrointestinal symptoms. The prevalence of CD in symptomatic patients and not-at-risk subjects was similar to that reported in Europe. Celiac disease appears to be a more common but neglected disorder than has generally been recognized in the United States.